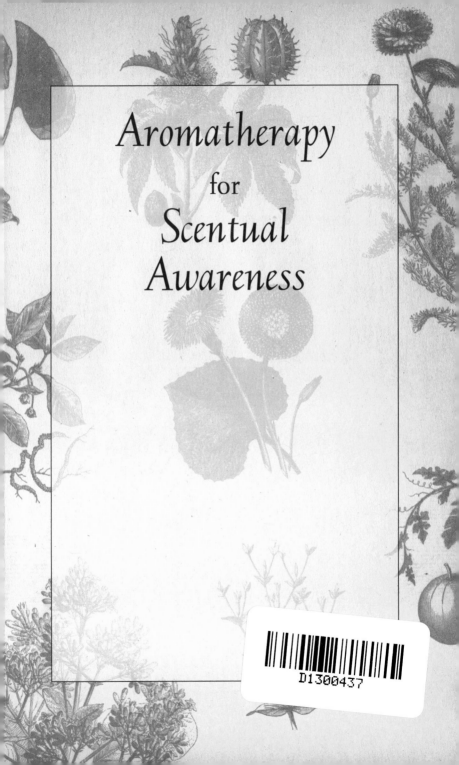

Aromatherapy
for
Scentual
Awareness

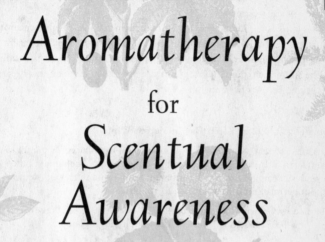

Aromatherapy

for

Scentual
Awareness

Care for the Body and Mind with
Nature's Essential Oils

Judith White and Karen Downes

Crown Trade Paperbacks *New York*

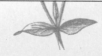

Aromatherapy is a natural therapy and a form of complementary medicine; however, it is strongly recommended that one should always consult a doctor before replacing any existing medication with an aromatherapeutic treatment. If you have any doubts about your health, consult your doctor before you embark on any treatment.

This book is not intended as a medical reference book. The information it contains is general, not specific to individuals. Do not attempt self-treatment for serious or long-term problems without consulting a qualified practitioner.

The authors and publishers disclaim all responsibility for any adverse reaction caused by use of essential oils.

Copyright © 1992 by Karen Day and Judith White

Published by Crown Trade Paperbacks, 201 East 50th Street, New York, New York 10022. Member of the Crown Publishing Group.

Random House, Inc. New York, Toronto, London, Sydney, Auckland

Originally published in Australia by Nacson and Sons Pty. Ltd. in 1992

CROWN TRADE PAPERBACKS and colophon are trademarks of Crown Publishers, Inc.

Printed in the United States of America

Design by Cynthia Dunne

Library of Congress Cataloging-in-Publication Data
White, Judith, aromatherapist.
    [Scentual awareness]
    Aromatherapy for scentual awareness : care for the body & mind with nature's essential oils / Judith White, Karen Day. — 1st ed.
    Originally published as: Scentual awareness. Brighton-Le-Sands, NSW : Nacson, 1992.
    1. Aromatherapy.   I. Day, Karen, aromatherapist.   II. Title.
RM666.A68W48   1996
615'.321—dc20   96-3808

ISBN 0-517-88666-9

10 9 8 7 6 5 4 3 2 1

First American Edition published 1996

*To our wonderful families who have
loved and supported
us every step of the way*

Acknowledgments

We give special thanks to James Burgin, our friend, for his ongoing motivation and support. To Leon Nacson, our devoted comrade, for his constant encouragement and confidence in us to write this book. To Arthur Stanley, wordsmith extraordinaire, for his creative insights. To Wendy Hubbert and Patty Eddy for taking this book beyond our Australian shores.

Contents

Introduction

WHILE WORKING WITH a group of students at the University of Wisconsin, Professor Arch Minchin uncovered what he and other scientists believed was a significant breakthrough in the study of olfaction—the sense of smell.

He found that by exposing his students to different aromas found naturally occurring in nature, under controlled conditions, he could substantially influence their moods and energy levels. Professor Minchin documented his findings and termed this phenomenon "scentual stimulation." It was scientific validation for what aromatherapists and numerous other natural therapists have known for years—that our bodies react strongly and impressively to different fragrances.

While science continues to try to unravel the mysteries behind our sense of smell, millions of laypeople are already tapping into the wonderful world of aromatics. How our olfactory receptor cells, located high in our noses, make sense of what they smell—discriminating infallibly between the fragrance of friends, the smell of newly cut lawn, a rose garden, burned toast, or a freshly brewed pot of coffee—is one of the great secrets of the world.

As people everywhere search for ways to improve the

quality of their lives in this sometimes unforgiving modern society, a greater awareness about the importance of staying in touch with nature is evolving. It is this very awareness that has led you to this book—and to us (Karen and Judith) putting pen to paper in the first place. We have spent the best years of our lives working with essential oils and applying them to people's individual needs. What we have witnessed, no scientist would ever be able to explain.

We have seen chronically ill people restored to health; we have seen sad and depressed men and women with a spring in their step for the first time in years; we have seen children's ailments clear up within hours; we have seen relationships blossom, love lives accentuated, and a general improvement in well-being and quality of life for tens of thousands of people—all through the use of aromatic essential oils.

That different blends of aromatic oils can elicit specific responses in the human body has engendered much disbelief and derision among many people not in touch with the workings and wonders of nature. Yet these oils—along with incense, perfume, and sweet-smelling herbs—have been used since time immemorial. When our ancestors were ill, they turned to the healing qualities of herbs and spices. They were inhaled, ingested, and worn as protective amulets. Egyptian priests of Cleopatra's time burned aromatics to help heal the sick, and when the Hebrews left Egypt, they took with them the formula for producing their aromatic medicines. Arab medicine in medieval times consisted of recipes using herbs, flowers, and spices to cure illness. When plagues raged through 17th-century Europe, which was beset by unsanitary conditions, hollow, fragrance-filled walking sticks and pomanders were carried, and the aromatics they contained were continually inhaled to ward off unpleasant odors and to protect against airborne infections. And during the reign of Charles II, bunches of rosemary were sold for the herb's healing qualities for six and eightpence.

There has rarely been a period, including our own, when odors and oils have not been important to the care of the body and mind. In fact, many of the essential oils that healed, soothed, and stimulated our ancestors are ingredients still employed by herbalists and modern perfumers.

Whether you realize it or not, the scents that surround you can change your mood, lift or lower your spirits, attract others to you, or put them off. They can energize or demoralize. As a matter of fact, sensory specialists have now established that smells can influence where you stand or sit in a room, how long you will stay, and how much you will enjoy yourself and the others in the room with you. Working and playing in a harmonious aromatic environment can instill confidence, help you concentrate, and give you a psychological edge.

There is an inner environmental revolution taking place, and at its center are our collective noses. Not since the early Egyptians have so many people recognized the importance of fragrance in helping us enhance our personal environments.

Air-cleansing machines have found a place in homes,

offices, and public spaces across the country. If we can't control the air in the outside world, we are determined to do something about the inner spaces around us. No wonder, then, that fragrance history has begun to repeat itself and that we are reevaluating the environments in which we spend our lives. All five senses are in full play, with emphasis on the most neglected—smell.

Like the citizens of every recorded society, we have turned to incense, potpourri, and pomanders to add to the quality of space we inhabit. Even today, people travel many miles just to sit and walk in a beautiful garden—just as they did in the days of the Gardens of Babylon. And why? Because it is instinctual that the very essence of nature is a healer to our spirit and to our soul. Of course our bodies respond to aromas! We don't need science to tell us that. Go sit in a beautiful garden and breathe in the brilliant blend of aromas, and you will notice an uplifting of your mood and spirit.

It is true, however, that some people respond more acutely and readily to aromas than others. This is not so unusual when you consider how magnificently developed the sense of smell becomes in a blind person. You can develop your senses far and beyond the average person's when you have to, or when you simply want to.

When women or men arrive at that stage of their lives when they become more aware of their senses, of nature and the world around them, we believe it marks a very important point in their development. *Scentual Awareness* is the term we use to describe this growing appreciation of aromas and fragrances, and the sense of smell—hence the title of this book. We believe our book can open the way to a whole new world for you. It will give you insight into a new approach to nature through one of its most powerful tools—the fragrant essential oils drawn from flowers and grasses, trees and roots, leaves and fruit. These remain the great untapped resources of our planet.

The following chapters will show you how each essential oil can offer many diverse benefits. You will see for yourself how aromatic oils can alleviate medical symptoms, prevent illnesses and disorders, influence our moods, or create special environments in our homes or offices—all without the chemical pollution of our bodies or our environment.

In writing this book, we have drawn largely on our own experiences in day-to-day life, in the visible improvements in our appearance, and in the general state of our health and well-being. We have also drawn on feedback from friends and relatives and, most important, from the thousands of people we have come in contact with through our work as aromatherapists, including many who have come to our workshops and demonstrations. They have all had stories to tell.

We invite you to follow us—and them—on this journey along the royal road to the subconscious, using the tried and tested blends of essential oils to evoke psychological and sensory responses. We want to share with you the secrets of an aromatic lifestyle that has transformed both of our lives.

We have a strong conviction that the solution to many of our common everyday ills and problems lies literally right under our noses, drawing us to them with their sweet-smelling aroma—nature's essential oils. These oils are intrinsic to our nature, which is akin to the alchemy of blending. Through aromatherapy, you can learn how to bring the essence of nature into your daily life.

1

Nature's Treasures

These are medicines which come out of the earth.
Mother nature has provided us with a complete
"materia medica."
　　　　　　—*The Family Herbal*, Dr. Peter Theiss

ESSENTIAL OILS MAY be used singly or in combination
to bring about curative and restorative processes in the
mind and body, offering a gentle alternative to medici-
nal drugs—many of which have horrendous side effects.

It is important, however, to understand that the
essential oils themselves *do not* cure. The body is the
hero when it comes to healing, and this is a basic principle and understanding of natural health. The essential
oils simply stimulate the already active healing, calming, and regenerative mechanisms within us.

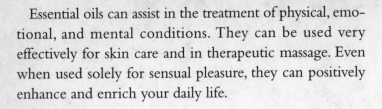

Essential oils can assist in the treatment of physical, emotional, and mental conditions. They can be used very effectively for skin care and in therapeutic massage. Even when used solely for sensual pleasure, they can positively enhance and enrich your daily life.

Since Time Immemorial

Some 2,000 years ago, the Father of Medicine, Hippocrates, recognized the value of aromatherapy when he spoke of the benefits of an aromatic bath and scented massage in restoring and maintaining physical and mental health. Even the biblical Scriptures speak of such healing power in the plant kingdom. Moses was directed to make a healing potion from "flowing myrrh, sweet cinnamon, calamus, cassia, and olive oil." Science has since established that such a potion has powerful antiviral and antibacterial properties. Myrrh is an effective antiseptic and its healing effects on open wounds, ulcers, and the like are well known.

Throughout the ages, men and women schooled in the various forms of medicine have recognized the tremendously powerful and diverse medicine cabinet that nature provides in its plant kingdom.

Aromatherapy

"Aromatherapy" simply means a therapy using aromas. The aromas come from the plant kingdom—flowers, trees, bushes, and herbs. The usual method of extraction is steam distillation, which produces a liquid with a distinctive fragrance and, in many cases, antiseptic, antiviral, and/or antibacterial properties, according to the individual plant. The relevant part of the plant—the wood of the sandalwood tree, the petals of the rose, the leaves of rosemary bushes, berries of the juniper tree—is put through this process of distillation, where the volatile, odoriferous substance is captured. It is this liquid that is known as the essential oil.

Essential oils evaporate quickly and are sensitive to both heat and light. This volatility varies from one oil to another, but, once bottled, essential oils will last for many years.

It is important to acquire only the purest essential oils, ones that have not been diluted or adulterated with any other oil or substance. Do not fall into the trap of buying cheaper, impure oils. Often they do not work effectively on a therapeutic level and there may be bodily reactions to the additives.

Unscrupulous suppliers will sometimes dilute a pure essential oil in a massage base oil and pass it off as pure natural essence. For this reason, it is advisable that you purchase your oils from a reputable company.

Essential oils need never be tested on animals. The most common method of testing is liquid gas chromatography, a proven scientific technique that identifies the active ingredients of each extract.

Essential oils have many uses, although our sense of smell, being so closely linked to our emotions, plays the largest part in recognizing the power of aromatherapy. We

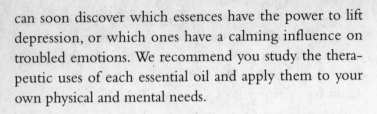
can soon discover which essences have the power to lift depression, or which ones have a calming influence on troubled emotions. We recommend you study the therapeutic uses of each essential oil and apply them to your own physical and mental needs.

True Natural Oils

Essential oils work quickly on both the body and the mind. Through our sense of smell, the olfactory nerves pass a message on to our brains, and scientists have shown that there is a physical and psychological response within four seconds. The essential ingredients of an oil are also absorbed quickly into the skin via the hair follicles, again with an almost instant effect.

Quality pure essential oils can be up to 70 times more concentrated than the plant source from which they are derived. The advantage of the natural product over a chemically created substitute is that the essential oil is more complex and retains all of its special properties.

You don't need vast experience as an aromatherapist to know a true essential oil when you come across it. The true natural oil stands out like the very nose on your face. Synthetically composed oils and perfumes made in a laboratory can never duplicate the transformation and life processes of nature.

Some philosophers believe that the aromatic flowering of plants is an offering to the gods from the plant kingdom. It is a beautiful offering when the plant is in its full manifestation or full bloom. Interestingly, the aromatic flowering is the last metabolic process the plant goes through before it starts its decaying process.

Synthetic vs. Natural

In perfumes and cosmetics, many hundreds of aromatic components are used, both natural and synthetic. These are blended accurately to maintain a consistent and stable product for a mass commercial market.

Within the world of aromatherapy, consistency of aroma is unimportant. The aromatherapist seeks out the highest-quality aromatic extracts from the plant to effect a healing response on the mind and in the body.

Essential oils will vary greatly in their chemical composition. Even some botanical species will differ in makeup when grown in separate locations or under variable growing conditions. Nature is ever-changing. This, of course, doesn't suit perfumers, so they include additives in their product to extend the natural aroma and maintain a constant floral bouquet.

With the development of technology, synthetic components become much cheaper, making production more economical. Synthetics or "aroma chemicals" are often said to be more durable, more economical, and more reliable than their natural counterparts; however, we must remember that they are not of the same making as essential oils.

Nature's laboratory allows a complex formulation to arise out of the plant—of the life force, some say. In the rich creation of the plant, a transformation of substance occurs and produces a direct link to our own design and makeup as a living organism.

Mother Nature brings to earth an abundance of life that provides the basis of existence for people and animals alike. The plant lives through light and through photosynthesis; its true characteristic is one of transformation. This process of transformation is an expression of life itself that cannot be copied, but it can be used as an energetic catalyst in our own bodies.

> *Seek out the very best oils for your individual needs. Accept only true and genuine natural plant extracts for a wholistic result and an aromatic experience.*

A synthetic fragrant product may have properties similar to a natural product, but this is not sufficient for an accurate qualitative assessment. The origin of the substance, as well as the process through which it was developed or obtained, is crucial to its quality and to the body's ability to assimilate and benefit from it.

Main Methods of Use

The two most common methods for using essential oils are vaporization and massage. Vaporization involves heating a few drops of your chosen oil in a ceramic vaporizer. The volatile elements of the oil evaporate into the air, and inhalation of the fragrance transfers the important molecules into the respiratory system.

When using an essential oil for massage, add a few drops to a good-quality "massage base" oil before use. Essential oils in the pure state are too highly concentrated to be used directly on the skin. The essential oils should be diluted in a base oil so that they can be massaged or rubbed onto the skin in the correct dosage. One drop of an essential oil may be all you need to use. When diluted in a base oil, it will cover a large area.

The best massage base oils are vegetable, nut, or seed oils (the vegetable oils used in aromatherapy should be cold-pressed). Some of the most popular base oils are outlined in Chapter 3, where we will expand on this theme of how to use the essential oils and give you a complete rundown on some of the ways these life-promoting substances are being used to great effect.

Effective Application

One of the other great advantages for turning to a true natural product for medical or cosmetic use is that the body has a greater affinity with natural ingredients and the oils can enter and leave the body with great efficiency, leaving no toxins behind.

The effectiveness of the skin in absorbing essential oils is well documented. Unlike chemical drugs, essential oils do not remain in the body. They are excreted through urine and feces, perspiration and exhalation. Studies show that expulsion takes 3 to 6 hours in a normal healthy body, and up to 14 hours in an obese or unhealthy one.

The healthier we are, the better we are likely to respond to the essential oils—and to any other natural therapy, for that matter.

Staying Healthy in Body and Mind

Essential oils can help us maintain harmony and balance in our lives, and promote better general health, a better appearance, and better all-around well-being.

But we must never overlook the basics of good health. No essential oil will help us if we do not look after our health in other ways. A healthy, nutritious diet, with a broad base of foods in their natural raw state, is essential. So are fresh air, sunlight (sunbathing, not sun baking), and exercise. Adequate rest and sleep are vital to allow our bodies time to recharge, regenerate, and renew. Rest and sleep are not the same thing. We need a good night's sleep and additional rest periods during the day.

Emotional poise is also important for our general health and well-being. Anyone who has ever gone through a broken relationship knows only too well the effects of stress. We have devoted an entire chapter to stress management and the emotions.

The essential oils can help us achieve our goals in all of these areas. They can stimulate or moderate our appetite, give us energy for exercise, promote restful sleep and slumber, and help balance our emotions.

2

The Aromatic Wardrobe

THE THIRTY ESSENTIAL OILS AND THEIR USES

Caesar's wife, Calpurnia, bathed in 20 pounds of crushed strawberries; Sarah Bernhardt took the plunge in champagne. Though generations apart, both were searching for what we all have at our fingertips today—luxurious treats for our physical and spiritual selves.

— From the Fragrance Foundation, London

WHEN WE SET out to put together a full complement of essential oils, we settled on thirty oils that we believe form the perfect aromatic wardrobe.

In essence, these oils make up a wonderful home health and beauty chest. The thirty oils we have included in our aromatic wardrobe give you great versatility. They will enable you to deal with a wide range of health complaints, as well as cater to all your skin and hair care needs. They will also provide support for your ever-changing emotional states.

This guide to the thirty essential oils will help you understand the vital characteristics of each oil so that you can judge for yourself how they can be used for better health and a more fulfilling life.

Basil
(Ocimum basilicum)

Basil is a pale yellow oil distilled from the leaves of the basil plant. It is an excellent all-around nerve tonic, an uplifting oil with a clarifying effect on the brain. It is extremely effective for relieving mental fatigue. Can be used in a vaporizer for mental concentration and decision making. Excellent for all kinds of respiratory ailments, such as bronchitis, and as a compress to relieve migraine headaches.

Benefits

Mind and Emotions—Focuses thoughts, promotes clear thinking and decision making.

Body—Antispasmodic, assists digestion, helps induce menstruation.

Skin Care—Stimulating tonic for congested skin (use sparingly), first aid for wasp stings and snakebites, mosquito repellent. Improves hair luster.

Conditions

    Colic, whooping cough, indigestion, migraine headaches, scanty menstruation.

Contraindications

    Do not use on the skin as a massage blend during the first three months of pregnancy.

Bergamot
(Citrus bergamia)

This delightfully fresh and citrusy essential oil is made by pressing the rind of a fruit resembling a miniature orange, which comes from the northern Italian town of Bergamo. Bergamot is an uplifting oil that helps to disperse anxiety or depression and relieve nervous tension. It blends well with other oils and has many uses. As a massage oil, it is an excellent acne treatment. It is also good for oily skin problems and dermatitis.

Benefits

    Mind and Emotions—Disperses nervous anxiety, uplifting, refreshing.

    Body—Stimulates appetite, antiseptic, relieves cramps.

    Skin Care—Assists healing (especially of eczema and dermatitis), highly antiseptic, cleansing.

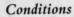

Conditions

Anorexia nervosa, stressful states, anxiety, eczema, dermatitis, intestinal parasites, adult colic, wounds and sores.

Contraindications

Berlock dermatitis. Not to be used externally in the presence of ultraviolet light, as with a tanning bed.

Cedarwood
(Juniperus virginiana)

One of the oldest known essential oils, Cedarwood may be used to relieve chronic anxiety and reduce stress. It is often used in men's toiletries. Cedarwood used in a vaporizer or inhaled is a great help with chest complaints such as catarrh and bronchitis. Used in conjunction with Rosemary, it can assist in restoring hair growth. Genuine Cedarwood essential oil has the fragrance of a freshly cut tree.

Benefits

Mind and Emotions—Releases long-term anxiety, relaxing, regenerating.

Body—Restorative, promotes longevity, relieves congestion.

Skin Care—Preserving, regenerating, hair restorer, relieves dandruff, psoriasis, eczema.

Conditions

Alopecia (hair loss), bronchitis, dermatitis, eczema, dandruff, psoriasis.

Chamomile (ROMAN)
(Anthemis nobilis)

Chamomile is a truly great essential oil. There are two main varieties: Roman and German. Both have similar properties, though Roman Chamomile has particularly calming, soothing effects on both the body and the mind. Used in a massage oil, Roman Chamomile is a good anti-inflammatory agent. It can be used in the treatment of skin allergies such as eczema. Roman Chamomile is especially good for balancing the female reproductive organs in a massage blend to the abdominal area. Chamomile is often used with children. Most people have at one time or another tried Chamomile herbal tea, a wonderfully calming and sleep-inducing drink. Chamomile and Lavender share some properties in common.

Benefits

Mind and Emotions—Relieves irritability, soothing, calming.

Body—Regulates menstruation, relieves painful menstruation, balances female reproductive system.

Skin Care—Deodorizing, relieves irritation, lightening to fair hair.

Conditions

Anemia, eczema, premenstrual tension (PMT), rheumatism, gout, flatulence, loss of appetite, conjunctivitis.

Chamomile (GERMAN)
(Matricaria chamomilla)

The most anti-inflammatory of all the essential oils, German Chamomile is a particularly good oil for massaging into inflamed tissue. It has wonderfully soothing properties and is extremely useful for inducing sleep and calming the mind and body.

Benefits

Mind and Emotions—Brings comfort, calming, gently sedating.

Body—Anti-inflammatory.

Skin Care—Relieves allergies, soothes dermal inflammation.

Conditions

Bursitis, hay fever, eczema, dermatitis, neuritis, neuralgia, thrush, abscesses, burns.

Clary Sage
(Salvia sclarea)

Distilled from flowers, Clary Sage has a sharp and slightly nutty aroma. This is the most euphoric of all essential oils. It is particularly effective in the types of stress-related problems many people experience. It helps to relax and uplift the most despondent person and relieve depressed thinking. It can be used as a compress and in a massage blend for general relaxation, and for the relief of menstrual pains.

Benefits

Mind and Emotions—Promotes communication, reduces tension (especially PMS), euphoric, uplifting.

Body—Regulates menstruation, relieves abdominal cramps, soothing to sore throats.

Skin Care—Antiwrinkle (especially older skins), cell regenerating, regulates production of sebum.

Conditions

Irregular and absent menstruation, abdominal cramps, premenstrual tension, frigidity, cellulite, depression, sore throat.

Cypress
(Cupressus sempervirens)

Cypress is distilled in France from the leaves and berries of the tree. Its woody fragrance is often used in men's toiletries. Cypress may help prevent asthma attacks. It is useful in the treatment of whooping cough and croup, all conditions where excess fluid is a problem. This highly astringent oil is ideal for treating oily skin.

Benefits
Mind and Emotions—Disperses nervous anxiety, relieves tension.

Body—Astringent, tonifying, vein tonic.

Skin Care—For oily skin, helps to strengthen veins, antiperspirant.

Conditions
Hemorrhoids, loss of voice, varicose veins, whooping cough, colds.

Eucalyptus
(Eucalyptus globulus)

There are many species of Eucalyptus. In aromatherapy, the leaves from Eucalyptus globulus are distilled to make the powerful Eucalyptus oil, which has a cleansing effect on the mind and body and a deodorizing effect on the environment. It is an excellent decongestant for colds and its antibacterial and antiviral properties can help stop the spread of infections and relieve the pain and itching of chicken pox, shingles, and cold sores. Use it in massage for arthritic pain or for muscular aches.

Benefits

Mind and Emotions—Invigorating, clarifying, energizing.

Body—Decongestant, relieves aches and pains, antiviral.

Skin Care—Promotes oxygen exchange, decongesting to sluggish skin, a good tonic.

Conditions

Respiratory disorders, sinusitis, high temperatures, rheumatism, coughs and colds, flu.

Fennel
(Foeniculum vulgare)

The oil is distilled from dried and crushed seeds of the Mediterranean plant. Fennel oil has a warm aniseed bouquet that is an ideal alternative to Peppermint. Fennel aids the digestive system, especially in the lower intestinal area. It relieves nausea, colic, and flatulence. It can help increase the flow of milk in nursing mothers, help relieve premenstrual tension, assist with weight loss, and decrease cellulite.

Benefits

Mind and Emotions—Calming, warming.

Body—Digestive support, balances estrogen, laxative.

Skin Care—Alleviates "orange-peel skin" associated with cellulite.

Conditions

Digestive problems, menopausal problems, obesity, constipation, nausea, flatulence, balances estrogen levels in the body.

Contraindications

Large doses can excite central nervous system.

Frankincense
(Boswellia thurifera)

The resin from which Frankincense is distilled has been burned on altars for centuries. Found now, as then, in Saudi Arabia and Somalia, it has a penetrating, soothing aroma. The effect of Frankincense on the mind and emotions is calming, and it is very useful for aiding meditation. It is an excellent oil to disperse fear, to fortify, and to comfort the spirit. Used as a skin tonic, Frankincense has a rejuvenating effect, especially for mature skins. It is an effective treatment for diarrhea.

Benefits

Mind and Emotions—Rejuvenating, comforting, fortifying.

Body—Deeply relaxing, heals old wounds.

Skin Care—Helps rejuvenate mature skin, healing, repairing.

Conditions

Sores, wounds, stress conditions, fear, nervous conditions, ulcerated skin, ulcers, diarrhea.

Geranium
(Pelargonium graveolens)

Helps balance mood swings, emotional highs or lows. It is the regulating oil to bring balance to hormonal change, as in menopause and puberty. The refreshing floral aroma relieves tension and is an excellent postbirthing choice for women.

Benefits

Mind and Emotions—Balances highs and lows, stabilizing, harmonizing.

Body—Balances hormones, regulates body functions, relaxing.

Skin Care—Promotes healing, normalizes sebum production, antiseptic astringent.

Conditions

Menopause, premenstrual tension, depression, mood swings, neuralgia, eczema, nervous tension, shingles.

Contraindications

Not to be used on inflamed and reddened skin.

Juniper
(Juniperus communis)

The Chinese revere the juniper tree for its immortal quality. The oil is distilled from ripe juniper berries, and has a fresh aroma. Juniper is an ingredient of gin and works to stimulate the appetite—hence gin and tonic as an aperitif. Juniper works on the mind to clear away unwanted emotions, thereby relieving tension. Its purifying effect brings relief for fluid retention and other toxic wastes, such as those connected with acne. This is the oil to relieve the symptoms of arthritis or bruising.

Benefits
Mind and Emotions—Reduces weepy emotions, purifying, clearing.

Body—Promotes cleansing, acts to tone the body and purify the blood.

Skin Care—Removes excess fluid, cleanses acne.

Conditions
Arthritis, rheumatism, gout, bruising, fluid retention, swelling, liver problems, obesity, general debility, urinary infections.

Lavender
(Lavandula angustifolia, Lavandula officinalis)

The best lavender grows on mountainsides in southern France. Probably the most popular and versatile essential oil, it has a soothing and calming effect, balancing and normalizing. It is an excellent first aid remedy. Lavender's properties range from antibacterial and cell stimulating to sedative and insect repellent. It may be used in a vaporizer, inhaled, applied neat on a small area or in dilution on a larger area. A highly active or restless child can often be calmed with just a few drops on the pillow. Lavender oil is excellent as a general tonic or during convalescence. It is strengthening and nurturing.

Benefits

Mind and Emotions—Gently sedating, nurturing and calming, soothing.

Body—Activates immune defense system, good for first aid, relaxing.

Skin Care—Cell rejuvenating, healing, soothes irritation.

Conditions

Infectious diseases, debility, scar tissue, heart conditions, hysteria, irritability, mosquito and other insect bites, dermatitis, burns.

Lemon
(Citrus limonum)

The light, clear, refreshing fragrance of Lemon uplifts the spirit and cleanses the mind. Lemon oil helps the body defend against infections, especially respiratory conditions. Used neat, it assists in the removal of warts. It is useful in the treatment of oily skin. This is one of the popular essential oils for children and the young at heart.

Benefits

Mind and Emotions—Increases mental alertness, refreshing and uplifting, clarifies thoughts.

Body—Respiratory and vein tonic, stimulating, clears the lungs.

Skin Care—Strengthens broken capillaries, nails, and hair, strengthens connective tissue, excellent as a tonic and astringent for oily skins.

Conditions

Dyspepsia, liver congestion, flatulence, gallstones, kidney stones, respiratory disorders, flu and colds, depression, mental fatigue.

Contraindications

Phototoxic, irritant when used undiluted, not to be used on skin in the presence of ultraviolet light, as with tanning beds.

Lemongrass
(Cymbopogon citratus)

Lemongrass, from which the essential oil is distilled, is often used in cooking. Lemongrass oil is toning and cleansing for the whole body. It is a fortifying oil that can help moderate nervous tension and anxious states. It is a powerful tonic and has a stimulating effect on the whole system.

Benefits

Mind and Emotions—Purifies the emotions, releases anxiety, nerve tonic.

Body—Cleanses and detoxifies, tones the muscles, antiseptic.

Skin Care—Stimulates the lymphatic system and reduces puffiness, helps reduce enlarged pores, strengthens connective tissue.

Conditions

Anxiety, colic, flatulence, muscle aches and pains, muscle and joint stiffness, obesity, stimulates milk supply.

Contraindications

Can irritate skin; use in low concentration.

Marjoram
(Origanum marjorana)

The warm, penetrating aroma of Marjoram works to lessen both physical and emotional responses. Its comforting properties help those who are suffering from grief, and its sedating qualities promote deep and restful sleep. It is an excellent massage oil for sore muscles and tension. Marjoram works as a sedative in a warm bath, and it blends well with Lavender.

Benefits

Mind and Emotions—Comforts grief, pacifying, deeply relaxing.

Body—Deeply sedating, relaxes muscles, antiaphrodisiac, relieves aches and pains.

Skin Care—Deeply relaxing.

Conditions

Sprains and strains, cramps, hyperanxiety, asthma, long-term insomnia, high blood pressure, bronchitis, grief, gout, moderates excessive sexual desire.

Contraindications

Not to be used on the skin as a massage blend during the first three months of pregnancy. Not to be used in the presence of low blood pressure or during times of depression.

Myrrh
(Commiphora myrrha)

This oil is renowned for providing courage and support for demanding physical and emotional performance. It is strengthening and rejuvenating. Myrrh is a very good expectorant and astringent, good for all kinds of coughs and colds. It may be used for gum disorders, and quickly heals mouth ulcers.

Benefits
Mind and Emotions—Inspirational, empowering for life's direction, fortifying.

Body—An expectorant, strengthening, soothing.

Skin Care—Cooling to wounds, rejuvenating to aged skin.

Conditions
Respiratory disorders, mouth ulcers, inflammation, diarrhea, bronchitis, wounds.

Neroli
(Citrus aurantium, amara)

This oil takes its name from an Italian princess who used it as her favorite perfume. Distilled from the flowers of the Seville orange, Neroli has a beautiful perfume, particularly when diluted. Especially useful in reducing states of anxiety, it can help in all kinds of stressful situations and can allay worries. It can sometimes assist in sensual arousal. By

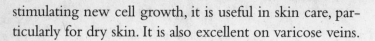

stimulating new cell growth, it is useful in skin care, particularly for dry skin. It is also excellent on varicose veins.

Benefits
Mind and Emotions—Calming, settling, sensual.

Body—Tonic for the heart, steadying during hormonal disturbances.

Skin Care—Vein tonic, strengthens capillaries, cell regenerating, soothing.

Conditions
Anxiety, hysteria, depression, nervous tension, insomnia, broken capillaries, sensitive skin, menopause.

Orange
(Citrus aurantium)

Distilled from the outer peel of the orange, this refreshing and uplifting oil blends well with others. Its energetic, refreshing fragrance promotes joyful communication. Orange used in a vaporizer is excellent for setting the mood for entertaining, especially when combined with Bergamot and Clary Sage. Orange is a gentle sedative and can help relieve acute headaches or mild insomnia. In skin care, it is useful for cleansing oily skin.

Benefits
Mind and Emotions—For joyful communication, exuberance, refreshing and uplifting.

Body—Relieves mild headaches, an "opening" oil.

Skin Care—Addresses open pores, softens hardened or cracked skin, allowing it to be cleansed, excellent for smoker's skin.

Conditions

Depression, anxiety, nervous conditions, constipation, muscular spasm, acute conditions, hysteria.

Contraindications

Not to be used topically in the presence of ultraviolet light, as with tanning beds.

Patchouli
(Pogostemon patchouli)

This oil has a rich Eastern aroma that can relieve anxiety and uplift despondent moods. Reputed to have aphrodisiac qualities that can be enhanced further by blending with Ylang Ylang. It works well as an antiseptic to heal chapped or broken skin and fungal infections, including athlete's foot. Old scar tissue responds well to a blend of Patchouli and Lavender.

Benefits

Mind and Emotions—Brings relief to anxious states, releases depression and lifts despondent moods, can enhance sexuality.

Body—Gentle antiseptic for open wounds, soothing to scraped and chapped skin, strengthening effect on tissue.

Skin Care—Regulates oil secretions, can be used to bring tone to slackened skin, helps repair scar tissue.

Conditions
Depression, anxiety, open wounds, tinea, diarrhea, acne, dermatitis, eczema, dry skin.

Peppermint
(Mentha piperita)

The fresh fragrance of Peppermint stimulates the mind and body to wakeful activity. Peppermint promotes clear thinking and stimulates the brain. It is energizing to the body when used as a massage blend. Peppermint aids digestion and has antispasmodic and analgesic qualities that relieve nerve pain. Inhaled directly, it clears the head and is an effective treatment for travel sickness and nausea.

Benefits
Mind and Emotions—Stimulates the mind, energizing, invigorating.

Body—The classic stomach remedy, stimulates digestion, settles upset stomachs, antispasmodic.

Skin Care—Cooling, decongestant for acne, rehydrating.

Conditions
Lethargy, indigestion, nerve pain, nausea.

Contraindications
Can cause skin irritation, use in low concentration.

Pine
(Pinus sylvestris)

Pine is the oil for inspiration. Inhalations of Pine are good for relieving colds and catarrh. A massage blend helps free chest and bronchials from the effects of colds, flu, and asthma. Pine has a stimulating effect on the circulation. It has a fresh aroma popular with most people, especially if working in air-conditioned environments.

Benefits
Mind and Emotions—Brings inspiration, clears the mind, refreshing.

Body—Stimulates circulation and oxygen exchange, expectorant.

Skin Care—Purifying, promotes oxygen intake.

Conditions
Respiratory problems, colds, catarrh, poor circulation, chest infections, rheumatism.

Rose Otto (ROSE)
(Rosa damascena)

The queen of all essential oils. The nurturing qualities of Rose Otto help mend emotional wounds, and bring physical and emotional stability. It uplifts depressed and despondent moods, and encourages fertility in women. Rose can balance the reproductive organs and is therefore an excellent choice for treating many health problems unique to women. Rose is the least toxic of all essential oils and will impart a healthy glow and vital appearance to the skin.

Benefits

Mind and Emotions—Balancing, rejuvenating, comforting.

Body—Promotes circulation, strengthens liver, balancing.

Skin Care—Cell regenerator, rehydrator, strengthens capillaries.

Conditions

For "broken hearts," depression, anxiety, hangovers, circulatory disturbances, menopause, frigidity, uterine imbalance, dry skin.

Rosemary
(Rosmarinus officinalis)

"Rosemary for remembrance." It is one of the most stimulating and awakening of essential oils, having a strong effect on the nervous system and acting as a brain stimulant to heighten sensory perception and memory recall. Rosemary is a good oil to use in massage, helping tired or injured muscles to recuperate. Traditionally used in hair care, mostly as a rinse or scalp rub, Rosemary can stimulate hair growth.

Benefits

Mind and Emotions—Memory activator, stimulating, enlivening.

Body—Enlivening to nervous systems, relieves muscular aches and pains, stimulates metabolism.

Skin Care—Antiseptic, cell regenerator, alleviates dry skin, dandruff, stimulates hair growth, adds luster to hair.

Conditions

Poor memory, lethargy, drowsiness, back pain, muscle aches, alopecia, baldness, gout, fatigue, sprains, obesity, liver congestion.

Contraindications

To be used with caution as a massage blend for those who have epilepsy.

Sage
(Salvia officinalis)

A highly antiseptic oil with a clean, sweet fragrance, Sage can be used to cleanse the mind and skin. It is best known for helping to normalize the body's intake and exchange of water. Sage is an excellent natural deodorant. It is also a calming oil with the ability to leave you with a sense of purpose and clarity.

Benefits

Mind and Emotions—Cleansing to thoughts, stimulating, refreshing.

Body—Antiseptic, cleansing, detoxifying. Kidney tonic.

Skin Care—Reduces puffiness, cleansing to oily skin, astringent, helps balance excess water or fluids in the body.

Conditions

Bacterial infections, rheumatism, excessive perspiration, sprains.

Sandalwood
(Santalum album)

Sandalwood is a strengthening aroma that brings courage and relieves irrational fears. It can have a stabilizing influence through many life changes. Long used as a perfume and incense, Sandalwood has a reputation as an aphrodisiac and for encouraging long bouts of sexual activity. As a cosmetic ingredient, Sandalwood aids the skin and has a pleasant aroma liked by both men and women. It has been used most successfully to bring relief to sore throats, laryngitis, and urinary tract disturbances.

Benefits

Mind and Emotions—Brings courage, helps to center and stabilize, strengthening.

Body—Kidney tonic, balances adrenals, useful at times of exhaustion, antiseptic.

Skin Care—Promotes elasticity, soothing to cracked or dry skin.

Conditions
Genitourinary problems, stressful situations, sore throats, skin infections, cystitis, depression, loss of courage.

Tea Tree
(Melaleuca alternifolia)

First aid in a bottle! Tea Tree oil has many uses and is active against bacteria, viruses, and fungi. A powerful oil, it should be used with caution at all times. Tea Tree oil can fight many infections, can assist in the removal of warts, and is effective in relieving the discomfort of bites, stings, boils, thrush, sore throats, sinusitis, cuts, and grazes. It is an excellent skin toner, especially for oily or infected skin.

Benefits
Mind and Emotions—Toning.

Body—Antiseptic, antifungal, antiviral.

Skin Care—Cleansing, disinfecting, antifungal, antibacterial astringent.

Conditions
Thrush, fungal infections, athlete's foot, acne, ringworm, mouth ulcers, herpes simplex, cysts, cystitis, sinusitis, bacterial infections, abrasions.

Contraindications
Keep away from eyes, keep away from children, use sparingly at all times.

Thyme
(Thymus vulgaris)

A fragrant culinary herb, Thyme is an antibacterial oil excellent for addressing respiratory, mouth, throat, and chest infections, topically. It works to stimulate the body's natural defense system, strengthening resistance to disease. Thyme's refreshing, herbaceous fragrance blends well with other oils, especially Lemon and Eucalyptus.

Benefits
Mind and Emotions—Energizing, activating, stimulating.

Body—Antiseptic, detoxifying, strengthens immune system.

Skin Care—Cleansing, antibacterial, purifying.

Conditions
Bacterial infections, colds, coughs, whooping cough, wounds, chest complaints, seborrhea, toxic conditions.

Contraindications
Mucous membrane irritant, do not use topically during pregnancy, avoid contact with the mouth and genital areas.

Vetiver
(Vetiveria zizanoides)

Vetiver has a deep, pungent aroma that brings strength and promotes the absorption and utilization of vital nutrients in the body. A relaxing oil, it helps release anger in ourselves and others. Vetiver is valuable as a bath oil and for use in massage, particularly related to stress. A useful skin-care aid for mature skin types, strengthening the deeper layers of the skin. It tends to draw possibilities and opportunities to you, and has been used throughout the ages to promote abundance and wealth.

Benefits
Mind and Emotions—Draws opportunities, promotes abundance, relaxing.

Body—Assists colon action, promotes healthy metabolism.

Skin Care—Regenerating at the deepest level, soothing to irritation, rejuvenating.

Conditions
Indigestion, intestinal disorders, long-term stress conditions, concern and worry, anger, constipation, premature aging.

Ylang Ylang
(Cananga odorata)

The exotic aroma of Ylang Ylang uplifts the spirit and dismisses anger at self and at others. This oil possesses warming qualities that promote sensual awareness and its aphrodisiac qualities can dissolve frigidity. Ylang Ylang is renowned for its settling effect on rapid heartbeat, and can help release depression. It blends well with Orange, Patchouli, and Sandalwood.

Benefits
Mind and Emotions—Sensual and exotic, uplifting, soothing.

Body—Aphrodisiac, cardiac tonic.

Skin Care—Helps balance combination skin.

Conditions
Tachycardia (racing heart), hypertension, depression, anxiety, oily skin, low libido.

Contraindications
Do not apply to inflamed skin, can cause headiness in high doses.

3

Aromatherapy in Action

Adrift in a warm and gentle sea of heavenly flowers, woods, herbs and spices.
—*Antony and Cleopatra*, William Shakespeare

THERE ARE MANY ways to use aromatherapy in your life. Here's how to get the essential oils working for you.

Bathing

There is something magical about immersing the body in warm, fragrant water. The benefits of aromatic bathing can be experienced at the end of a tiring day when you need to relax and release the tensions that have built up. Aromatic oils can also be used beneficially at the start of the day to invigorate and refresh you after sleep.

The aromatic scenting of waters is a custom that has been observed for centuries. Used primarily to wash and perfume the body, essential oils made cleanliness easier for our ancestors because of their antibacterial properties.

Bathing with essential oils stimulates the opening of congested pores and can release muscle tension and fatigue. To pamper yourself, simply fill a bathtub with water, close the bathroom door, and create an ambience suitable to your mood, perhaps with candlelight. Dispense 6 to 8 drops of oil into the bathwater and agitate the surface to disperse the molecules. Use one favorite oil or your personal blend of up to three essential oils. Relax in the bath immediately to take advantage of the warm and fragrant vapors. Spend 15 minutes soaking. When leaving the bath, pat your skin lightly, leaving a fine layer of the essential oils on the skin surface for further absorption.

If your tub is big enough, there is no better way to unwind with your partner at the end of a busy day than by sharing an aromatic bath.

The essential oils will be beneficial to your mind and emotions through your sense of smell, and beneficial to your body by absorption through the skin.

ESSENTIAL OIL COMBINATIONS FOR THE BATH

To Relax

Orange—2 drops	*Sandalwood—2 drops*
Patchouli—4 drops	

To Uplift

Bergamot—5 drops   Ylang Ylang—1 drop
Orange—2 drops

To Sedate

Lavender—2 drops   Sandalwood—2 drops
Marjoram—3 drops

To Invigorate

Lemon—2 drops   Rosemary—3 drops
Pine—3 drops

To Harmonize

Cedarwood—2 drops   Lavender—3 drops
Geranium—2 drops

Vaporization

You can make your home or work environment more relaxing or uplifting by using a vaporizer.

Vaporization provides the perfect means to permeate the atmosphere with the delightful aromas of pure essential oils. As the droplets evaporate into the air, our sensitive olfactory nerves transmit the scent to our brains. The effect on our minds and bodies starts within seconds.

The ideal way to vaporize essential oils is to use a ceramic vaporizer. A few drops of the chosen oil (or a combination) are placed in a shallow dish filled with water on the top of the unit. A small candle that can last 6 to 8 hours is lit underneath the dish. The heat from the candle gently evaporates the water and oils together into the surrounding air.

The oils in the air also provide an extremely effective antiseptic air freshener. Vaporizers assist breathing by helping to relieve the respiratory imbalances of asthma or croup. You can use an uplifting oil to aid concentration at home or at work, or to set the scene for a wonderfully intimate evening with your partner.

All of the aromatic wardrobe essential oils are suitable for vaporization. But it is important that you choose oils that you like and that are pleasing to the senses. Just as some essential oils can have a positive influence on your moods and emotions, if you don't like the oil being vaporized you may notice your mood slipping a little.

You will find that by varying the oils and combinations, you will be able to change the atmosphere in your surroundings. You can choose when to relax or stimulate your senses, and when to refresh and uplift weary spirits. There are oils to sedate and help you sleep and oils to calm the overactive child or adult.

It is always best to blend your own aroma, choosing the oils you feel happiest with at a particular time. Of course, you must first get in touch with all the essential oils from your aromatic wardrobe so that you know which ones to use.

☙ **Dinner Parties.** An ideal combination to set the mood for a social event is 3 drops each of Orange and Clary Sage oils and 2 drops of Peppermint oil in a vaporizer. Very uplifting!

❧ **Meditation.** Five drops of Myrrh, 3 drops of Frank-incense, and 2 drops of Pine oil make a peaceful, spir-itual blend suitable for meditation and inspiration.

❧ **Partytime (for children).** A lighthearted blend that will set a fresh, cheerful mood at a child's party con-sists of 5 drops of Orange oil and 3 drops of Lavender.

❧ **Room Freshener.** A good all-purpose room fresh-ener can be made from 3 drops each of Lemongrass and Eucalyptus oil, and 2 drops of Sage oil.

❧ **Mood Elevator.** Two drops of Orange oil, 4 drops of Clary Sage, and 2 drops of Neroli provide an effective way to raise flagging spirits.

Massage

If there is another method of using the essential oils that rivals the luxurious bath for sheer pleasure, it is massage. Who doesn't enjoy a good, soothing massage? Massage is such an important subject that, in Chapter 10, we will show you various massage techniques for specific pur-poses such as relief of pain and tension, general well-being and communication, or sensual massage with a special partner.

The aromatic massage can be as professional or as per-sonal as you like; the rubbing action will activate the nerve endings in your body and stimulate the circulation of blood to the surface of the skin, thereby increasing the absorption of the oils into your body. Massage has an incredibly relaxing effect on the body in its own right.

Combined with aromatherapy, it becomes a powerful therapeutic tool.

To relax and tone the body, add aromatherapy massage to your daily routine. Massage is so important—it promotes circulation, stimulates the release of toxins through the lymphatic system, and provides a sense of warmth and well-being. As the body is cleansed of toxins, the skin is given a new suppleness and elasticity.

We firmly believe that we all need to experience and share touching to maintain our emotional and physical balance. Up to three or four essential oils can be combined with a massage base oil to incorporate the individual expressions of each oil, working together to produce the most effective results.

MAKING YOUR OWN BLEND

Blending your own massage oil can be part of your aromatherapy ritual. This also gives you the freedom to choose different oils for your massage. By blending only small quantities, you will also maintain your oil's freshness, and by personalizing your blend, you will maintain your own quality control. Blending each day lets you create a "day by design."

MASSAGE FOR OTHERS

Using aromatherapy massage with others is a beautiful way to share a sensory experience. The combined effect of the massage and the essential oils can heighten sensual awareness, relax, or stimulate, according to your moods and the oils you use.

MASSAGE FOR YOURSELF

Massage is usually thought of as being applied by another person, but it is not always possible to share the massage experience with a partner. Don't ignore the pleasures and benefits of self-massage. Take time to massage your own body from head to toe and renew your own body awareness.

Nurturing and caring for yourself will increase your self-esteem and your sense of self-worth. It can also make you more attractive to others. The sensory experience of using essential oils enhances awareness and will turn a normal, everyday activity into a joyous, aromatic, and sensual experience.

Select your own personal blend of oils to suit the activities of the day to come. For example, use Basil and Rosemary to stimulate and aid concentration, Lavender and Bergamot to soothe and calm.

The letting-go of physical tensions during massage often stimulates the release of emotional tension. The cumulative effects of massage are very strong and promote a lasting feeling of well-being.

MASSAGE BASE OILS

Essential oils in the pure state are too highly concentrated to be used directly on the skin, and you will therefore find references to massage base oils (sometimes known as carrier oils, or base oils) throughout the book. The essential oils are diluted in a base oil so that they can be massaged or rubbed onto the skin in the correct dosage.

Massage base oils are vegetable, nut, or seed oils, many of which themselves have therapeutic properties. Base oils are obtained from the seeds of plants that grow all over the world. There are several hundred different plants known to have oil-bearing seeds, but only a few have been produced commercially. Base oils are usually produced for food and therefore are good sources of nutrients and energy.

Before we give you a rundown of the important massage base oils, there are some important points to remember when using these oils for your massage blends.

- *The oils should always be cold-pressed so as to retain vitamins and minerals.*

- *Oils should be stored in glass containers, preferably amber or blue glass.*

- *In hot, tropical climates it is a good idea to keep them in the refrigerator until shortly before they are to be used.*

- *Many base oils turn rancid after a period of time and should be used within twelve to eighteen months. Macadamia and jojoba, which can last for eight to ten years, are the exceptions.*

Body Massage Oil—Sweet Almond Oil

This is a light, fine, odorless oil ideal for general massage. It is traditionally used to prevent skin from wrinkling, and has a high nutritional value. It helps relieve itching, soreness, dryness, and inflammation.

Facial Skin Oil—Peach Kernel Oil

A fine-textured oil, rich in vitamins, and one of our favorites for body and especially facial massage, it is often used in warm oil treatments with the addition of essential oils. Peach Kernel is excellent for dry or sundamaged skin, and has long been used by Chinese women to refine their skin texture.

Warming Body Oil—Olive Oil

This base oil has a wonderfully warming effect on the whole body. It is particularly good for children, the elderly, and those who acutely feel the cold. It is also a valuable scalp and hair tonic. A wonderful base oil to address cellulite, with the addition of essential oils.

Nourishing Body Oil—Avocado Oil

A highly penetrative oil, used on its own as a luxury base or combined with sweet almond. It is excellent for dehydrated skin types. It is rich in vitamins A and E and ideal for expectant mothers to help prevent stretch marks.

Vitamin Oil—Wheat Germ Oil

This oil is high in vitamin E. A 10 percent addition of this oil to a massage base such as sweet almond will help to preserve your blended oils. An excellent oil for the treatment of eczema or dermatitis, and also very good for healing burns.

Wheat germ oil is rarely used on its own, but is a valuable addition to other base oils.

Luxurious Body Oil—Jojoba Oil

A natural fluid wax, nongreasy, and quickly absorbed by the skin, jojoba oil acts as a luxurious moisturizer for aging, dry, and hardened skin types. It leaves your skin with a beautiful silky softness, and will not turn rancid. It is a superb base for massage and hair treatments.

Balancing Body Oil—Evening Primrose Oil

A superb base oil. It contains gamma linolenic acid, vitamins, and minerals, and is often recommended by doctors and naturopaths as a dietary supplement. It is excellent in the treatment of psoriasis, and helps to prevent premature aging of the skin.

Rejuvenating Body Oil—Macadamia Nut Oil

Extremely high in vitamin A, this oil, with its warm, nutty aroma, promotes rejuvenation. An excellent body oil for daily skin care to nourish and moisturize, it is highly valued for its antioxidizing properties.

Here's one of our favorite recipes for a luxurious massage blend of cold-pressed oils.

Macadamia oil—77 percent   Jojoba oil—10 percent
Avocado oil—10 percent   Essential oil blend—3 percent

Enjoy!

PREPARING YOUR MASSAGE OIL

To prepare your massage oil, pour 10 milliliters (⅓ fluid ounce) of the chosen massage base oil into a small glass or glazed ceramic bowl (never use plastic containers for essential oils). Add 5 drops of the essential oil or a blend of up to three oils of your choice, then apply to the body.

General Rule: Whatever the number of milliliters of massage base oil, you should add half that number of drops of essential oil. If you have 10 milliliters (⅓ ounce) of massage base oil, you should add 5 drops from your chosen blend of essential oils.

This amount of base oil will be sufficient for a fine layer over the skin, although you may need 1 full ounce for a large and/or hairy person. Make sure to apply only the finest layer so that the skin glows and is not greasy. Continue to rub it in until absorbed. Your oil blend should be left on the skin after massage to be absorbed into the body.

Inhalation

Inhalation is another way in which vaporization of essential oils is used to balance physical disorders and help release emotions.

Take a stainless steel or glass bowl and fill it halfway with near-boiling water. Have ready your chosen oils and a towel. Add a few drops of oil to the water, and agitate gently to release the vapors. Close your eyes, and breathe deeply over the bowl with the towel over your head. Continue for up to 10 minutes for maximum benefit.

Suggested Combinations and Uses

- **Sinusitis.** You can relieve sinusitis by using 2 drops each of Peppermint and Eucalyptus oils in a vaporizer or by inhaling them from a handkerchief.

- **Bronchial Congestion.** To ease bronchial congestion, inhale 2 drops each of Eucalyptus and Cedarwood oils from a handkerchief or steam bowl, or use in a vaporizer.

- **Releasing Fears.** Three drops of Frankincense and Myrrh oil in an inhalation will help release feelings of fear.

- **Relieving Mental Fatigue.** Two drops of Basil and 2 drops of Rosemary in an inhalation will bring mental clarity and stimulate memory.

_____ **Compresses** _____

There are two specific uses for a compress. For facial skin care, it is useful for softening the skin and promoting cell regeneration. For therapeutic applications, compresses may be used in first aid. They can help relieve pain and swelling, and will reduce inflammation. Hot compresses are generally used to relieve chronic pain, while cold compresses are ideal for acute pain or injury.

You can also release pent-up emotions by inhaling the vapors from a warm aromatic compress. Fold a piece of sheet or toweling to make your compress, then soak it in hot or cold water to which a few drops of an essential oil have been added. Make sure the cloth absorbs as much of the oil as possible from the surface of the water.

FACIAL COMPRESS COMBINATIONS

For Mature, Dry Skin

Clary Sage—1 drop   Sandalwood—2 drops
Frankincense—1 drop

For Oily Skin

Cypress—2 drops   Lemon—2 drops

First Aid Compress *(for bruising/swelling)*

Frankincense—1 drop   Lavender—2 drops
Juniper—1 drop

For Period Pains/Premenstrual Tension

Basil—2 drops   Clary Sage—2 drops

For Facial Neuralgia

Peppermint—3 drops

There are many other methods of use for the essential oils, particularly in the areas of skin and hair care. We'll look at these more specific beauty treatments a little later.

ANTIWRINKLE LOTION

Drop 20 rose petals into 10 fluid ounces of boiling water and allow to infuse for 10 minutes. Remove the petals and add 1 drop of Rose essential oil and 1 drop of Frankincense. Shake vigorously and keep well sealed when cooled. Use on a pure cotton pad to wipe over the face and throat area. This lotion is balancing to dry skin and regenerating to mature skin types. Use night and morning after cleansing the skin.

How to Use Your Essential Oils: A Summary

❧ **Bath.** Add 6 to 10 drops of essential oil to a full bath. Agitate the water to disperse the oil evenly before entering the water. Warm water to relax, and hot to revitalize.

❧ **Blend.** Use a 1:2 ratio of essential oil to massage base oil—that is, 5 drops of essential oil to every 10 milliliters (⅓ ounce) of base oil. Store in a dark glass bottle with a tight lid.

❧ **Compress.** Disperse 3 to 6 drops of essential oil or a blend of oils into a half pint of water. Agitate the water for thorough oil dispersion. Place a cloth or gauze square on top of the water, then place the fabric on the affected area. When using the compress to soak the skin, as in your skin care program, fully immerse the cloth in the aromatic water.

🌿**Douche.** Add 5 drops of essential oil to 1 pint of tepid water.

🌿**Flavorings (culinary use).** Essential oils may be added to food preparations. Remember, these oils are highly concentrated, so be sparing. Only 1 or 2 drops are required, such as 1 drop of Lemongrass onto a teabag to make a full pot of tea.

🌿**Foot Bath.** Disperse 6 drops of essential oil into a large bowl of warm to hot water. Agitate the water. For foot massage treatment, place a cloth in the bottom of the bowl and drop a few large marbles on top of the cloth. Roll the marbles around with the soles of your feet. Take a footbath at mealtimes, late in the evening to help you relax, or after a hard day at work. Soak the feet for a minimum of 15 minutes.

🌿**Inhalation.** Use 3 to 4 drops of an essential oil or blend of oils in a bowl of near-boiling water. Place a towel over the head and bowl and inhale gently. This is an invaluable aid in relieving mental fatigue or colds, flu, and sinus congestion. Alternatively, add 1 to 2 drops of oil neat onto a handkerchief.

🌿**Perfume.** Apply a few drops of essential oil onto the palm of your hand. Rub your hands together and quickly run your fingers through your hair. Or add oils to a cotton pad and place within your clothing. You can blend two or three different oils to make your individual scent.

Spray/Spritz. Use a blue glass bottle or stainless steel spray can. Fill with distilled or purified water. Add 3 to 4 drops of essential oil and agitate. Use as a facial toner, spritz to refresh skin, room freshener, or treatment for animals or plants. *Note:* Never use plastic containers for essential oils.

Swab (direct application). Apply a few drops neat onto a cotton ball or a sterile gauze pad, and apply to the affected area. When using the compress to soak the skin, as in your skin care program, fully immerse the cloth in the aromatic water.

Vaporization. This method can be used to create the perfect atmosphere for any occasion. You can select oils that will help you relax, revitalize, work, rest, or play. Take a ceramic vaporizer and fill the bowl on top with water. Light the candle in the base. Disperse 6 to 8 drops of your chosen essential oil in the water. As the water warms, it releases healing vapors into the air.

Wash/Swab. Disperse 3 to 6 drops of essential oil into 6 ounces of distilled or purified water. Agitate the water. Bathe the desired area with aromatic water and a cotton pad. When storing your aromatic wash, do so in glass bottles and change regularly, about once a week.

4

Aromatic Dressing

We live our lives focusing primarily on the external world. The source of our power, to live a vital energetic life, comes from within. It's time to consciously embrace our internal mechanics, which nourish the soul and drive our actions.

—Judith White

NATURAL OILS HAVE always been the backbone of the cosmetic industry's most successful products. Throughout history, all the beauties have used oils. Some bathed in them. Others massaged them into their skin.

Oils protect and moisturize the skin; when used regularly, they give the skin a sheen that catches the light and makes heads turn.

"Aromatic dressing" is the term we use to create a day by design. It involves a daily body rub with essential oils, which will nourish the skin and the underlying tissue and organs. This aromatic action will also embrace the way you feel and think as part of your daily skin care and beauty regime.

We firmly believe that aromatic dressing is the secret to staying vital and energetic throughout your life. As you nourish and protect your skin daily with selections from your aromatic wardrobe, the skin will reflect a healthy glow while maintaining a constant state of well-being.

Every morning we go to our wardrobe to select clothing for the day. We make our choices based on the weather, the day's appointments, comfort and color, our feelings—the list goes on. Individual expression has as big a role to play in our choices as the need for suitable warmth and protection.

With your aromatic oils, you can make similar decisions. Every morning after showering, you can select from your aromatic wardrobe to dress your body's needs—from the inside out.

We suggest choosing three essential oils to combine into a base oil, creating an aromatic blend. Once you familiarize yourself with the essential oils, you can make your decisions based on how you want to feel for the day ahead—physically, mentally, and emotionally—be it for a business meeting, a sports event, lunch with a friend, a day with the children, or a sensual evening with your lover.

There are so many variations you can concoct with the essential oils that you will be able to find a perfect combination that moisturizes your skin and makes it look and feel great, and appeals to your nose and aesthetic judgment as well.

Giving Yourself the Best Possible Start to the Day

Morning. It is that very special time of the day that can determine just how you function throughout the next 24 hours. By being positive and ensuring that you have a healthy, invigorating start, you really are giving yourself the best possible chance of a successful day ahead.

These are our favorite morning regimes, using the essential oils to enhance the appearance and lift the spirits. Take it from us, they work!

Morning Option I
(On Rising)

Step 1

Light your oil vaporizer. Select an oil to invigorate your body and activate your mind.

Frankincense—to rejuvenate.
Lemon—to uplift.
Peppermint—to invigorate and motivate.
Rosemary—to stimulate and activate.

Step 2

If possible, walk barefoot into the back/front yard. Experience your feet on the earth, grass, soil, or sand. Take in the sky, nature, and your surroundings. Breathe in the essence of the morning. Breathe deeply and release three times. Communicate with the seasons and connect with yourself as part of the universe.

Step 3

Do some stretching, then commence a morning walk. Studies have shown that regular physical activity can help to overcome or reduce depression and fatigue. Regular aerobic exercise pumps up vitality, improves muscle tone and circulation, and detoxifies your body.

Walk at a brisk pace, pumping the arms, for 30 to 45 minutes every day—or you can make your walks part of our recommended rotation system of exercise (see Chapter 11).

Step 4

Time to cleanse with a brisk body polish in the shower. With the skin dampened, add a few drops of one of your morning oils to 6 ounces of warm water. A blue or amber glass bottle will hold your aromatic splash and enable you to agitate the water and oils easily. Sprinkle over the upper body and begin to brush with a natural bristle body brush in a to-and-fro motion to polish your body. Move from the hands to shoulder girdle, over the chest and rib cage. Use circular rotations in a rhythmical action over the abdomen and the buttocks. Move down the spine and across the back, then down the legs to the feet. Focus on the soles of the feet to stimulate the circulation.

Step 5

Pat your skin dry. Take a ceramic or glass vessel to create a blend from your aromatic wardrobe for the day ahead.

Pour in your base oil and add the essential oils. Begin your body rub. Smooth a small amount of oil over the skin and briskly rub your blend into the skin so that it glows and is not greasy. You can apply your blend to the face as well as the whole body.

Step 6

Robe your body for 15 minutes, allowing the oils to deeply penetrate into the body via the hair follicles.

Morning Option II
(On Rising)

Step 1

Light your vaporizer. Select an oil to invigorate your body and mood to prepare for the day ahead.

Eucalyptus—to clarify and invigorate.
Geranium—to balance and harmonize.
Orange—to uplift and refresh.
Sandalwood—to strengthen and encourage.

Step 2

Breathing exercise—to enhance lung capacity and embrace the day. Inhalation/exhalation—the intimate exchange between our outside world and our inside world. A rhythmical connection between our conscious and subconscious.

Resting your hands on your rib cage at your sides just above the waist, breathe out completely. Now inhale gently through the nose, letting your abdomen swell as much as it will to a count of four. Let your ribs and then your chest expand under your hands (don't raise the shoulders). Hold your breath for a count of eight and then let it out through your mouth as you count slowly to four, noticing how your rib cage shrinks beneath your hands and pulling in with your abdomen until you have released as much air as possible and tightly contracted your abdominal muscles. Repeat four times.

Step 3

Your body is now ready to be cleansed, awakened with stimulation, and rejuvenated. Take your body brush into the shower along with your aromatic splash (see step 4, Morning Option I). Once the body is wet, sprinkle a few drops of aromatic water over the damp-ened skin and begin body brushing. Using long sweep-ing strokes, begin with the arms and move over the shoulders and down to the fingertips, paying attention to the hands. Sweep over the chest and around the breast and rib cage, using circular rotations over the abdominal area.

Work your brush over the back, on either side of your spine. Move onto the buttocks, using firm circu-lar movements and sweeping strokes up and down the entire leg to move surface lymph, which detoxifies the body. Pay attention to the toes and feet to remove any calloused skin. Dry your body.

Step 4

Choose a beautiful bowl or vessel in which to create your aromatic blend. Add your chosen cold-pressed base oil and personal blend. With circulation stimulated, the body is warm, ready to receive your essential oils. Massage the oils over the entire body so that the skin is glowing, not greasy.

Your body and mind are now awakened and ready for a well-earned breakfast to further sustain the body.

Bathing Ritual

In ancient times, priests would cleanse and anoint themselves daily as an act of dedication to pure thoughts and ideals. The Greeks introduced bathing for inner and outer therapy, while the Romans brought bathing to the height of total personal pampering. Great public baths became luxurious spas for cleansing, scenting, and socializing.

You can add this quality of richness and rejuvenation to your daily program to enhance the quality of your sensory experiences and heighten your state of bliss. We believe it is essential to complete one "cell renewal" bath per week, as follows:

1. Warm the bathroom area and fill your tub with warm-to-hot water. Have towels and robe ready.

2. Prepare your signature blend of oil in a medium-sized ceramic vessel. Make sure you are seated in a comfortable position.

3. Smooth the oil over your skin lavishly, from the toes to the upper chest area. Take a body brush and dip into your blend.

4. Begin with small circular movements over the hands, arms, shoulders, chest area, abdomen, toward the pelvis and buttocks. Move down the legs and embrace the feet.

5. Once the entire body has been covered you are ready to immerse yourself in your bath. Soak for 10 to 15 minutes in warm water.

6. Leave the water and pat the skin dry. Your body will feel alive and your senses aroused. Robe yourself to keep warm.

_____ The Perfect Close to Your Day _____

Create an aromatic environment that enhances a mood of peace and calm. Light a candle, adorn a small area with flowers, and choose your oils for the day's end. Ignite your vaporizer and find space to lie down and begin your deep breathing, to discover and reconnect with your body, to release emotional or physical tensions, or to experience heightened sensual awareness.

_____ Suggested Evening Blends _____

Deep Sleep

Lavender—2 drops   Orange—2 drops
Marjoram—4 drops

Sweet Dreams

Cedarwood—2 drops Orange—4 drops
Lavender—2 drops

Restful Slumber

Cedarwood—3 drops Sandalwood—3 drops
Lavender—2 drops

Forty Winks

Lavender—2 drops Neroli—3 drops
Marjoram—3 drops

Sensuous Breathing

Lie on the floor on your back and relax as much as you can, letting your body "melt away" into the floor, allowing your arms and legs to flop. Close your eyes and feel your body against the floor, paying special attention to any tension points in any part of your body. Just be aware.

Now focus inside your body and ask yourself where you feel any sensation in your muscles because of your breathing. Anywhere you feel tense, imagine you are breathing into that spot. Imagine you can exhale through that part of the body and, as you do, experience the breath relaxing sore muscles as it filters through them.

Now that you are relaxed, you can experiment with the beautiful movements that are part of natural free breathing. When you breathe in, feel your pelvis tip back gently so there is a slight arch to your back while your abdomen and chest rise, ribs and back expand, and chin tilts forward. Then, when you exhale, your pelvis moves down again so your spine almost touches the floor, your back contracts, and your chin and head move back again, exposing the front of your neck a bit more. This natural movement is a wavelike motion that flows without hesitation from each in-breath to its following out-breath and so on. Practice. Exaggerate the tiny movements at first until you get the feel of it, then it will flow naturally.

This is a wonderful ritual to do outdoors.

Daily Use of Essential Oils

Personally, we both have a deep sense of commitment to aromatherapy—and we are sure that you too, if you haven't already, will soon enjoy using the essential oils as part of your daily health and beauty regime.

There are all sorts of ways you can incorporate the oils into your life. On rising, you can follow one of the wonderful morning regimes we have documented earlier in this chapter or make up your own program. You may choose a combination of oils that stimulates you physically, or one that is cleansing and refreshing.

Giving your body a wet-skin brush while under the shower is an excellent way to cleanse the skin, get rid of old skin cells, and stimulate circulation. We feel that dry-skin brushing can be too harsh.

Family members can have a great time contributing to the family aromatic environment at mealtimes or on other occasions. We sometimes keep aromatic diaries in our homes for weeks at a time. You can use these diaries to write special messages to your loved ones. A good idea for a special person is to add 1 drop of a particularly well-liked oil to the sheet of paper on which you are writing a personal message.

Your car is another great place to use aromatic oils. We regularly put a drop of our favorite oil onto a tissue and tuck it into the air vent ducts. You can then enjoy an aromatic journey. You can use the oils in your workplace, too. Both at home and at work, we have facecloths in our bathrooms with a selection of essential oils so that everyone can refresh themselves with a hot aromatic inhalation as they wash off their face and hands. We also carry facecloths and our essential oils in our handbags so we can refresh ourselves throughout the day, no matter where we are.

When we go to our respective homes at night, we always light our vaporizers and use oils to relax and unwind. We usually like to take aromatic showers before retiring, or soak in a tub with a few drops of oil. If we've been on the go all day, we like to restore our feet in a revitalizing footbath and sit with our children while they eat their dinner. The vapors come up from under the table and delight us all.

The gym is another place where you can use the essential oils. In our lockers at the gym, we each have our own complement of oils. You can make your own steam room and sauna environment. Having a body rub after your workout with a blend of oils is heaven on earth!

We encourage you to use the essential oils as your first choice when reaching for a household remedy, or when a mood enhancer is needed in social or business situations. The possibilities are limitless, and you will find by trying the different oils that some suit you more than others. The secret is to experiment and enjoy awakening your own senses and those of your friends and family.

Here are some great recipes to help you incorporate the oils into your everyday life.

The Fundamentals

RELAX AND REVIVE

The Relaxation Kit

Bergamot, Cedarwood, Lavender

For calming, balancing, and uplifting. Use in your bath.

SUCCESS WITHOUT STRESS

The Office Kit

Basil, Lemon, Rosemary

For stimulating productivity and clear thinking. Use in a vaporizer.

ESSENSUALITY

The Romance Kit

Orange, Patchouli, Ylang Ylang

For sensuality, sexuality, and soothing. Use in a vaporizer.

SKINSENSE

The Massage and Skin Care Kit

Sweet Almond Base Oil
Cedarwood, Frankincense, Geranium

For relaxing, regenerating, and fortifying.

INNER PEACE

Meditation Kit

Frankincense, Myrrh

For connecting with your higher self and clarifying life's direction. Use in a vaporizer.

Needless to say, we love aromatherapy. We live it. We breathe it. We invite you to tap into this delightful source of joy and nourishment. We guarantee that if you do incorporate the oils into your daily regime, you will see noticeable changes in your life.

Skin: The Body's Largest Organ

Before we show you what oils to use on different parts of your body, it is important that you understand how your skin works and how best you can protect it.

Few people realize that the skin is the largest organ of the body. In a person weighing about 165 pounds, the skin constitutes approximately 6⅔ pounds, whereas the liver is a mere 3⅓ pounds. The skin is only about .04 to .08

inch deep on most areas of your body, although on the palms of the hands and soles of the feet it is thicker—about .16 inch.

Skin is composed of three distinct layers: the outer epidermis, the only part we see, which is continually renewing itself as new cells are formed and old ones are shed from the surface; a deeper layer called the dermis, which contains the connective tissue that lends skin its remarkable strength, suppleness, and pliancy; and the subcutaneous tissue, which is responsible for nourishing and insulating us.

The skin is endowed with a very good supply of blood, brought to the surface by tiny capillaries. It is also teeming with nerve endings, which are responsible for our perception of touch and pain.

One of the skin's main functions is the elimination of wastes, sweat, and excess sebum, the lubricating oil produced by the sebaceous glands. These are excreted through tiny pores that cover the entire surface of the skin. Oxygen and carbon dioxide also pass in and out of the skin, in a kind of respiration akin to that which takes place in the lungs.

Some people argue that the skin doesn't absorb much of the essential oils, but this is patently untrue. Essential oils have the ability to penetrate right into the deep layers of the skin, and from there they travel to the various organs, glands, and tissues of the body. Once they have passed through the epidermis, they seep into the small capillaries in the dermis and are carried all around the body in the blood. They are also taken up by the lymph fluid, which bathes every cell in the body.

A simple test you can carry out on yourself, which shows just how effectively essential oils are absorbed and transported around the body, is to rub the soles of your feet with a clove of garlic. A few hours later, you will be able to smell garlic on your breath. This is why an ancient remedy for colds and respiratory infections is to put garlic in your shoes.

Similarly, many modern medicines—particularly those for seasickness and travel sickness—come as patches that stick onto your skin, usually on the neck area. The medication is absorbed through the skin and into the blood.

So let's now have a look at how the essential oils can be used to improve your health and well-being and your appearance.

5

Health and Healing

There is a remedy for every illness to be found in nature.

—Hippocrates

NATURAL HEALING RECOGNIZES that the human body is superbly equipped to resist disease and heal injuries. But when disease does take hold, or an injury occurs, the first instinct is to see what might be done to strengthen the body's natural resistance and healing agents.

The ancient Greek physician Hippocrates (460–377 B.C.), considered to be the father of modern medicine, was an advocate of essential oils as a way of stimulating the body's own healing mechanisms. He taught the healing properties of many plants and herbs and actively encouraged their use.

But even though plants and plant essences featured strongly in all ancient forms of medicine, it was not until early in this century that a French scientist, R.-M. Gattefossé, coined the term *aromathérapie*—by which he meant the therapeutic use of odoriferous substances, obtained from flowers, plants, and aromatic shrubs, through inhalation and application to the skin.

Marguerite Maury, a biochemist and one of the pioneers of aromatherapy, has described the aromatic extracts of plants as the "purest form of living energy that we can transfer to man."

_____ Treating Illness _____

Simple. Effective. Safe. More and more people these days are looking to natural therapies as an alternative to conventional medicine and its unwanted side effects.

We know from years of experience that aromatherapy can be used to treat most common ills very effectively. Studies suggest that aromatic oils work by stimulating the body's own healing mechanisms, often bringing about a quick therapeutic response. There is nothing mysterious about this process. Herbs—many of which have similar properties to the essential oils we mention in this book— are routinely used by medical doctors in Europe and elsewhere—as a safer alternative to drugs.

We believe essential oils are one of the most powerful natural healing modalities of this time. They work in perfect balance, addressing the threefold aspects of the human being as a whole—body, mind, and emotions. Essential oils work on the subtle life energies of the human organism. They promote a feeling of well-being that permeates the conscious and physical components of the body, establishing a "eubiotic" or balancing effect, reducing the degree of imbalances, if and when they occur.

Acupuncturists, acupressure therapists, and others who work with touch for health have learned to love essential oils because they know that these oils can have strong effects on the meridians within the body. These therapists believe oils can balance excess and low energies and provide them with an additional tool with which to reestablish balance in the body.

We routinely use essential oils to treat ourselves and our children. Friends and family members have benefited from our knowledge, too. We have heard from countless clients how various oils have worked wonders on their health problems.

Aromatherapy can be used not only to treat illness effectively, but also to prevent us from losing our good health in the first place. Today, we must be in action to stay well. Many of us live and work in large cities where pollution and emotional stress levels can take a toll on our health. More and more women pursue careers—often on top of running a home and looking after a family—which put demands on them that were largely unknown even fifty years ago. Indeed, the many stressors of modern living can diminish the energy reserves needed to maintain health.

Of course, we do not wish to turn back the clock, and it would be foolish to refuse to accept all the technological advances of the modern world. We have to adapt ourselves to cope with the ever-changing modern environment, and this is where aromatherapy is so helpful. By inhaling the essences and massaging plant oils into the skin, we firmly believe you can build up natural resistance to stress and illness. We want to encourage you to spend your valuable time enjoying and celebrating life, rather than nursing physical or emotional disease.

In a way, aromatherapy can provide us with many of nature's gifts that we miss by living in cities and towns, as it re-creates the fragrances of the trees and the flowers that would naturally surround us in the country.

We invite you to try aromatherapy as your first-choice treatment for common ills and injuries. Of course, this isn't to say that proper medical diagnosis shouldn't be sought and, where needed, conventional treatment applied. But as your confidence in the powers of aromatherapy grows, you may find that trips to the doctor and your local pharmacy become less frequent.

The recipes in the following section on aromatherapy treatments have been specially formulated from years of research. We have continually refined these recipes according to our vast clinical and personal experiences. They are, therefore, very effective. Use them with confidence.

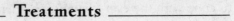

Treatments

ABRASIONS AND CUTS

Lavender, Patchouli, Tea Tree, distilled water

Antiseptic Wash

Lavender—2 drops	Tea Tree—2 drops
Patchouli—2 drops	Distilled water—3 ounces

It's important to keep the skin clean and bacteria-free when it is injured.

ABSCESS

Chamomile (German), Lavender, Tea Tree, base oil

Antiseptic Swab

Chamomile—1 drop	Tea Tree—1 drop
Lavender—1 drop	

Place 3 drops onto gauze or cotton pad and dab on.

ALLERGIES AND HAY FEVER

Chamomile (German), Geranium, Lavender, base oil

Soothing and Calming Massage Blend

Chamomile—10 drops	Lavender—22 drops
Geranium—13 drops	

It is vital to isolate any irritating agents. Make time to soothe away emotional and physical discomfort.

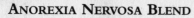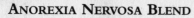
ANOREXIA NERVOSA BLEND
Bergamot, Clary Sage, Geranium, Rose Otto, base oil

Appetite Stimulant

Bergamot—13 drops   *Geranium—15 drops*
Clary Sage—17 drops

Body Rebalancer

Clary Sage—20 drops   *Rose Otto—8 drops*
Geranium—17 drops

These are massage blends. It is important to counter the desire to lose weight.

ANXIETY
Basil, Bergamot, Cedarwood, Geranium, Lavender, Lemongrass, Sandalwood, base oil

Soothing (nervous butterflies)

Basil—8 drops   *Lavender—17 drops*
Bergamot—20 drops

Strengthening (chronic anxiety)

Cedarwood—17 drops   *Lemongrass—8 drops*
Lavender—20 drops

Calming (acute anxiety)

Geranium—8 drops   *Sandalwood—17 drops*
Lavender—20 drops

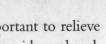

These are all massage blends. It is important to relieve feelings of uneasiness and tension and provide a relaxed, nurturing, and comforting state of being.

ARTHRITIS (RHEUMATISM)
Chamomile (German), Eucalyptus, Frankincense, Juniper, Lavender, base oil

Joint Repair

Eucalyptus—10 drops	*Juniper—10 drops*
Frankincense—10 drops	*Lavender—15 drops*

Add German Chamomile when acute inflammation is present. You can use this massage blend to ease any joint inflammation that may cause pain or lead to restriction of movement.

ASTHMA
Eucalyptus, Juniper, Lavender, Marjoram, base oil, hot water

Breathe–Easy Massage Blend I *(for children or in acute adult conditions)*

Eucalyptus—15 drops	*Lavender—20 drops*
Juniper—10 drops	

Breathe–Easy Massage Blend II *(for adults or in chronic cases)*

Eucalyptus—15 drops	*Marjoram—10 drops*
Lavender—20 drops	

Breathe-Easy Inhalation Blend *(for clearing the sinuses)*

Eucalyptus—2 drops   Marjoram—1 drop
Lavender—1 drop

These blends will help you to maintain ease of breathing, free from restriction. Pure essential oils will assist in opening air pathways, offering immediate relief.

ATHLETE'S FOOT

Eucalyptus, Lavender, Pine, Tea Tree, Thyme, base oil

Antifungal Swab

Eucalyptus—1 drop   Tea Tree—1 drop
Lavender—1 drop

Using a cotton ball, dab onto the skin.

Antifungal Massage Blend

Pine—15 drops   Thyme—15 drops
Tea Tree—15 drops

BITES AND STINGS

Lavender, Lemongrass, Peppermint, Tea Tree, base oil

Bite and Sting Swab

Lavender—1 drop   Tea Tree—1 drop

Dab with a cotton ball or swab.

Repellent Blend

Lavender—20 drops   *Peppermint—10 drops*
Lemongrass—15 drops

To be used topically.

BOILS

Chamomile (German), Lemon, Lavender, Thyme, distilled water

Antiseptic Swab

Chamomile—1 drop   *Lavender—1 drop*

Dab onto cotton ball and onto skin.

Cleansing Wash

Lemon—2 drops   *Thyme—1 drop*
Lavender—3 drops

Pour into 3 ounces of water.

BREAST MASSAGE BLEND COMBINATIONS

Chamomile (Roman), Cypress, Fennel, Geranium, Juniper, Lavender, Lemon, Lemongrass, Peppermint, Rose Otto, Sage, base oil, cold water

Toner

Cypress—10 drops   *Sage—20 drops*
Lemon—15 drops

Enlarger

Fennel—20 drops   Rose Otto—10 drops
Geranium—15 drops

Reducer

Cypress—20 drops   Lemon—15 drops
Juniper—10 drops

Nipple Ease *(for nursing mothers)*

Rose Otto—5 drops   Jojoba oil— $\frac{1}{3}$ ounce

Be sure to thoroughly remove the massage blend from the nipple area prior to feeding your baby.

Anti-inflammatory Compress

Geranium—1 drop   Rose Otto—1 drop
Lavender—2 drops

In cold water.

Engorgement Relief

Geranium—30 drops   Peppermint—15 drops

Milk Reducer

Cypress—20 drops   Sage—25 drops

Milk Producer

Fennel—30 drops   Lemongrass—15 drops

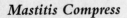
Mastitis Compress

Geranium—1 drop   Peppermint—2 drops
Lavender—2 drops

In cold water.

BRONCHITIS

Cedarwood, Eucalyptus, Lavender, Marjoram, Pine, Tea Tree, base oil, hot water

Relief Inhaler

Eucalyptus—2 drops   Marjoram—1 drop
Lavender—1 drop

Acute Bronchitis Massage Blend

Eucalyptus—15 drops   Tea Tree—15 drops
Lavender—15 drops

Preventive Massage Blend

Cedarwood—15 drops   Pine—10 drops
Eucalyptus—20 drops

Chronic Bronchitis Massage Blend

Cedarwood—10 drops   Marjoram—10 drops
Eucalyptus—10 drops   Tea Tree—15 drops

BRUISES

Cypress, Juniper, Lavender, base oil, cold water

Soothing Swab

Cypress—1 drop   Lavender—1 drop

Repair Massage Blend

Cypress—10 drops   Lavender—20 drops
Juniper—15 drops

Repair Compress

Cypress—2 drops   Lavender—3 drops

BURNS

Lavender, base oil, cold water

Lavender Swab

Lavender—2 drops

Apply with a cotton ball.

Lavender Spray

Lavender—4 drops

After-Sun Massage Blend

Lavender—45 drops

CATARRH

Cedarwood, Eucalyptus, Juniper, Lemon, Peppermint,
Pine, base oil, hot water

Expectorant Massage Blend

Cedarwood—10 drops   Lemon—10 drops
Eucalyptus—15 drops   · Pine—10 drops

To be applied topically.

Breathe-Easy Inhaler

Eucalyptus—2 drops *Pine—1 drop*
Peppermint—1 drop

Breathe-Easy Massage Blend

Cedarwood—10 drops *Juniper—10 drops*
Eucalyptus—15 drops *Peppermint—10 drops*

To be applied topically.

CELLULITE

Fennel, Juniper, Lavender, Rosemary, base oil

Anticellulite Massage Blend

Fennel—10 drops *Lavender—10 drops*
Juniper—10 drops *Rosemary—15 drops*

Daily massage with this blend will assist in the removal of cellulite from the body tissue. However, diet and exercise must also be addressed.

CHICKEN POX

Chamomile (German), Lavender, Tea Tree, base oil

Relief Blend

Chamomile—10 drops *Tea Tree—15 drops*
Lavender—20 drops

CHILBLAINS

Chamomile (German), Juniper, Lavender, Rosemary, Sandalwood, base oil, warm water

Soothing Massage Blend

Chamomile—15 drops   Lavender—30 drops

Soothing Footbath

Chamomile—2 drops   Lavender—4 drops

Prevention Rub

Juniper—15 drops   Sandalwood—20 drops
Rosemary—10 drops

CHILDBIRTH CONDITIONS

Bergamot, Cedarwood, Clary Sage, Frankincense, Geranium, Lavender, Marjoram, Orange, Sandalwood, jojoba base oil

Perineum Massage

Jojoba oil

Pregnancy Blend

Bergamot—10 drops   Lavender—20 drops
Cedarwood—15 drops

Prebirth Blend

Frankincense—15 drops   Sandalwood—10 drops
Orange—20 drops

First-Stage-Labor Blend

Bergamot—10 drops   Lavender—20 drops
Clary Sage—15 drops

Second-Stage-Labor Blend

Lavender—15 drops   *Sandalwood—10 drops*
Marjoram—20 drops

Postlabor Blend *(antidepression blend)*

Clary Sage—15 drops   *Lavender—20 drops*
Geranium—10 drops

These are all massage blends.

CIRCULATION

Bergamot, Cedarwood, Eucalyptus, Lavender, Lemon,
Lemongrass, Marjoram, Peppermint, Rosemary, Sage,
Sandalwood, Tea Tree, base oil

High Blood Pressure Blend

Cedarwood—10 drops   *Marjoram—20 drops*
Lavender—15 drops

Low Blood Pressure Blend

Bergamot—15 drops   *Sandalwood—10 drops*
Rosemary—20 drops

Stimulating Blend

Eucalyptus—10 drops   *Rosemary—15 drops*
Lemon—10 drops   *Sage—10 drops*

Midwinter Blend

Eucalyptus—15 drops   *Rosemary—10 drops*
Peppermint—10 drops   *Tea Tree—10 drops*

Lymphatic Cleanser Blend

Eucalyptus—10 drops   Lemongrass—15 drops
Lemon—10 drops   Rosemary—10 drops

These are all massage blends.

COLDS AND FLU

Basil, Cedarwood, Eucalyptus, Lemon, Marjoram, Peppermint, Pine, Tea Tree, Thyme, base oil, boiling water

Sinus Relief Inhaler

Eucalyptus—2 drops   Tea Tree—2 drops
Peppermint—2 drops

Cough Relief Massage Blend

Basil—10 drops   Peppermint—10 drops
Eucalyptus—15 drops   Pine—10 drops

Can be applied topically.

Daily Comfort Massage Blend

Eucalyptus—15 drops   Pine—10 drops
Lemon—10 drops   Tea Tree—10 drops

Can be applied topically.

Nighttime Bath

Eucalyptus—3 drops   Pine—2 drops
Marjoram—2 drops   Thyme—1 drop

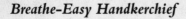

Breathe-Easy Handkerchief

Eucalyptus—2 drops   *Pine—2 drops*
Peppermint—2 drops

Apply neat onto a handkerchief and inhale throughout the day.

Expectorant Massage Blend

Cedarwood—15 drops   *Lemon—10 drops*
Eucalyptus—15 drops   *Pine—5 drops*

Can be applied topically.

Colds discharge unwanted waste from the body, so the aim of the treatment is to gently restore health and vitality, rather than suppressing the symptoms of the illness.

COLD SORES

Eucalyptus, Geranium, Lavender, Myrrh

Cleansing Swab

Eucalyptus—1 drop   *Myrrh—1 drop*
Lavender—1 drop

Fragrant Lipstick

Eucalyptus—1 drop   *Geranium—1 drop*

Drop onto the back of the hand or into a small dish. Apply lipstick to lipstick brush and mix with the essential oils. Apply to lips in the usual manner.

COLIC

Basil, Chamomile (Roman), Lavender, Marjoram, Peppermint, base oil

Baby Colic Blend

Lavender—30 drops

Children's Colic Blend

Chamomile—15 drops   *Lavender—30 drops*

Adult Colic Blend

Basil—10 drops   *Peppermint—15 drops*
Marjoram—20 drops

These are all massage blends.

CONJUNCTIVITIS

Chamomile (Roman), cool water

Eyewash

Chamomile—2 drops

Shake well into 3 ounces of cool water, let stand 24 hours before using. This is excellent for relieving sore, red, inflamed, strained, and puffy eyes.

CONSTIPATION

Fennel, Lavender, Lemongrass, Marjoram, Rosemary, base oil

Children's Blend

Lavender—15 drops   *Rosemary—15 drops*
Marjoram—15 drops

Adult Blend (acute)

Lemongrass—15 drops   Rosemary—15 drops
Marjoram—15 drops

Adult Blend (chronic)

Fennel—10 drops   Rosemary—20 drops
Lemongrass—15 drops

These are all massage blends. Massage abdominal area and lower back in a clockwise direction.

CONVALESCENCE

Clary Sage, Geranium, Lavender, base oil, warm water

Restorative Bath

Clary Sage—2 drops   Lavender—4 drops
Geranium—2 drops

Restorative Massage Blend

Clary Sage—15 drops   Lavender—20 drops
Geranium—10 drops

CORNS

Lavender, Lemon, Orange, very warm water

Softening Footbath

Lavender—2 drops   Orange—2 drops
Lemon—2 drops

Soak feet for at least 15 minutes.

CROUP

Eucalyptus, Juniper, Lavender, Marjoram, olive oil base

Breathe-Easy Massage Blend

Eucalyptus—15 drops   Lavender—10 drops
Juniper—10 drops   Marjoram—10 drops

Breathe-Easy Steam Room

Eucalyptus—5 drops   Lavender—5 drops
Juniper—5 drops   Marjoram—5 drops

The Breathe-Easy Steam Room is great for children and adults who suffer from croup or asthma. Cover the shower drain and turn on the hot water, adding drops of oil to the running water. Steam for ten minutes.

CYSTITIS

Cedarwood, Cypress, Frankincense, Juniper, Lavender, Sandalwood, Tea Tree, base oil, warm water.

Cystitis Blend (acute)

Frankincense—10 drops   Sandalwood—10 drops
Juniper—10 drops   Tea Tree—15 drops

Apply topically.

Cystitis Blend (chronic)

Cypress—10 drops   Sandalwood—10 drops
Juniper—10 drops   Tea Tree—15 drops

Apply topically.

Calming Bath

Cedarwood—2 drops   Sandalwood—3 drops
Lavender—3 drops

DEPRESSION

Basil, Bergamot, Clary Sage, Neroli, Patchouli, Sandalwood, Ylang Ylang, base oil

Uplifting Massage Blend *(acute)*

Basil—10 drops   Neroli—10 drops
Bergamot—15 drops   Patchouli—10 drops

Antidepressant Massage Blend *(chronic)*

Clary Sage—15 drops   Sandalwood—10 drops
Neroli—10 drops   Ylang Ylang—10 drops

These mixtures will help relieve depression by working on an emotional level. Essential oils affect us both emotionally and physically as they enter the olfactory system. They can quickly elevate withdrawn states.

DERMATITIS AND ECZEMA

Bergamot, Chamomile (German), Geranium, Lavender, Patchouli, Sandalwood, base oil

Dermatitis Blend

Bergamot—15 drops   Lavender—20 drops
Geranium—10 drops

Dermatitis Blend No. 2

Bergamot—10 drops   Lavender—15 drops
Chamomile—10 drops   Sandalwood—10 drops

Dry Eczema Blend

Bergamot—15 drops   Sandalwood—10 drops
Lavender—20 drops

Wet Eczema Blend

Lavender—20 drops   Sandalwood—10 drops
Patchouli—15 drops

These are all massage blends.

DIAPER RASH

Lavender, base oil

Everyday Basic Massage Blend

Lavender—30 drops
Sweet almond oil—2 ounces

Everyday Luxury Massage Blend

Jojoba oil—3 ounces   Lavender—30 drops

DIARRHEA

Cypress, Fennel, Lavender, Patchouli, base oil

Regulating Blend (acute)

Cypress—15 drops   Patchouli—15 drops
Lavender 15 drops.

To be applied topically.

Regulating Blend *(chronic)*

Cypress—10 drops   Lavender—10 drops
Fennel—10 drops   Patchouli—15 drops

To be applied topically.

DIGESTION

Basil, Fennel, Peppermint, base oil

Digestive Aid

Fennel—25 drops   Peppermint—20 drops

Indigestion Relief

Basil—10 drops   Peppermint—20 drops
Fennel—15 drops

Our fast lifestyles, rapid eating, and irregular meals can play havoc with digestion. Massage daily for optimum health, or use these oils in your vaporizer.

EARACHE

Lavender, Peppermint

Chronic Earache Swab

Lavender—1 drop   Peppermint—1 drop

Place on a small swab of cotton and apply just inside the ear.

ECZEMA

See Dermatitis and Eczema.

EDEMA

Chamomile (German), Frankincense, Juniper, Lavender, base oil

Dispersion Massage Blend

Chamomile—10 drops   Lavender—15 drops
Juniper—20 drops

Dispersion Compress

Frankincense—1 drop   Lavender—1 drop
Juniper—2 drops

EYES (sore, red, inflamed, strained, puffy)

See Conjunctivitis.

FAINTING (lightheadedness)

Peppermint, Rosemary, Sandalwood, base oil

Grounding Massage Blend

Peppermint—10 drops   Sandalwood—20 drops
Rosemary—15 drops

Use topically for frequent fainting. (You should, of course, consult your physician if this condition persists.) If fainting occurs infrequently, use the blend on a tissue to breathe in.

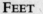

FEET

Peppermint, Rosemary, Sage, base oil, hot water

Reviver Bath

Peppermint—2 drops   Sage—2 drops
Rosemary—2 drops

Reviver Massage Blend

Peppermint—10 drops   Sage—15 drops
Rosemary—20 drops

Odor-Eater Footbath

Sage—6 drops

Relaxing the soles of the feet can bring immediate relief to many discomfort zones in the body.

FEVER

Eucalyptus, tepid water

Relief Compress

Eucalyptus—4 drops

Relief Bath

Eucalyptus—8 drops

FLATULENCE

Fennel, Lavender, Lemon, Lemongrass, carrier oil

Abdominal Blend *(acute)*

Fennel—20 drops   *Lemongrass—10 drops*
Lemon—15 drops

Abdominal Blend *(chronic)*

Fennel—10 drops   *Lemon—15 drops*
Lavender—20 drops

Use these blends topically. Naturally, dietary changes can also be made. Regular exercise and emotional poise are also important.

FRACTURES

Lavender, Rosemary, Sandalwood, Thyme, base oil

Bone Repair Massage Blend

Lavender—10 drops   *Sandalwood—15 drops*
Rosemary—10 drops   *Thyme—10 drops*

FRIGIDITY

Clary Sage, Geranium, Lavender, Orange, Rose Otto, Sandalwood, Ylang Ylang, base oil

I'm Safe Massage Blend

Clary Sage—10 drops   *Lavender—15 drops*
Geranium—10 drops   *Rose Otto—10 drops*

Sensual Massage Blend

Orange—15 drops   *Sandalwood—10 drops*
Rose Otto—10 drops   *Ylang Ylang—10 drops*

Use these blends topically.

FUNGAL INFECTIONS
See Athlete's Foot; Yeast Infection.

GASTRITIS
Basil, Chamomile (German), Chamomile (Roman), Fennel, Lavender, base oil

Child's Massage Blend

Chamomile (R)—15 drops   *Lavender—20 drops*
Fennel—10 drops

Adult's Massage Blend

Basil—15 drops   *Fennel—20 drops*
Chamomile (G)—10 drops

GINGIVITIS
Cypress, Lavender, Myrrh, Tea Tree, toothpaste, warm water

Mouthwash

Cypress—1 drop   *Tea Tree—1 drop*
Lavender—1 drop

Add these oils into ⅓ glass of warm water and vigorously rinse the mouth, agitating the water back and forward through the teeth. Spit it out when finished.

Aromatic Toothpaste

Myrrh—1 drop	*Tea Tree—1 drop*

Drop oil onto toothpaste and apply with brush.

GOUT
Basil, Fennel, Juniper, Rosemary, base oil

Antigout Massage Blend

Basil—10 drops	*Juniper—15 drops*
Fennel—10 drops	*Rosemary—10 drops*

GUMS (sore, infected, bleeding)
See Gingivitis.

HAY FEVER
Cypress, Eucalyptus, Lavender, Marjoram, base oil, hot water

Breath-Easing Inhalation

Cypress—1 drop	*Lavender—1 drop*
Eucalyptus—2 drops	

Chest Rub

Eucalyptus—10 drops	*Marjoram—10 drops*
Lavender—25 drops	

HEADACHES

Basil, Chamomile (Roman), Lavender, Marjoram, Orange, Peppermint, Rose Otto, Rosemary base oil, hot water

Clear-Head Blend

Chamomile—1 drop   Orange—2 drops
Lavender—3 drops

Use hot water as an inhalation.

Chronic Headache

Inhale   **Massage Blend**
Basil—3 drops   Basil—15 drops
Orange—1 drop   Orange—10 drops
Rosemary—1 drop   Rosemary—10 drops
Rose Otto—1 drop   Rose Otto—10 drops

Migraine Headache

Inhale   **Massage Blend**
Basil—1 drop   Basil—10 drops
Marjoram—3 drops   Marjoram—15 drops
Peppermint—1 drop   Peppermint—10 drops

See also Migraine.

HEMORRHOIDS

Cypress, Lavender, base oil, warm water

Sitz Bath

Cypress—2 drops   Lavender—3 drops

Massage Blend

Cypress—20 drops   Lavender—25 drops

HYPERACTIVITY AND HYPERTENSION

Bergamot, Lavender, Marjoram, Orange, sweet almond base oil

Daytime Massage Blend

Bergamot—15 drops   Marjoram—10 drops
Lavender—20 drops

Nighttime Bath Blend

Lavender—2 drops   Orange—2 drops
Marjoram—4 drops

INDIGESTION

See Digestion.

INFLUENZA

See Colds and Flu.

INSOMNIA

Lavender, Marjoram, Orange, base oil, warm water

Massage Blend

Lavender—20 drops   Orange—15 drops
Marjoram—10 drops

Evening Bath

Lavender—4 drops   *Orange—2 drops*
Marjoram—3 drops

Sleepy-Time Pillow Swab

Lavender—2 drops   *Orange—1 drop*
Marjoram—3 drops

Drop onto cotton pad and place inside pillowcase.

JET LAG

Lavender, Rosemary, Sandalwood, Ylang Ylang, jojoba
base oil

Preflight Massage Blend

Lavender—30 drops   *Ylang Ylang—15 drops*

In-Flight Blend

Lavender—2 drops   *Ylang Ylang—1 drop*

Place on hot, wet facecloth and wipe over face and
neck.

On Arrival Bath *(daytime)*

Rosemary—4 drops   *Sandalwood—4 drops*

On Arrival Bath *(nighttime)*

Lavender—3 drops   *Ylang Ylang—2 drops*
Sandalwood—3 drops

LABOR

See Childbirth Conditions.

LARYNGITIS

Clary Sage, Cypress, Sandalwood, Tea Tree, base oil

Throat-Ease Massage

Clary Sage—10 drops   Tea Tree—15 drops
Sandalwood—20 drops

Throat Swab

Clary Sage—1 drop   Sandalwood—1 drop

Apply drops neat to throat. Take care.

MASTITIS

Chamomile (German), Eucalyptus, Geranium, Lavender, Rose Otto, tepid water

Soothing Bath

Chamomile—4 drops   Rose Otto—2 drops
Lavender—2 drops

Soothing Compress

Eucalyptus—2 drops   Lavender—1 drop
Geranium—1 drop

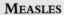

MEASLES

Chamomile (Roman), Eucalyptus, Lavender, tepid bath water

Soothing Bath

Chamomile—2 drops   Lavender—4 drops
Eucalyptus—2 drops

MENSTRUATION

Basil, Bergamot, Chamomile (Roman), Clary Sage, Eucalyptus, Geranium, Lavender, Peppermint, Rosemary, Rose Otto, base oil

PMS Blend

Clary Sage—15 drops   Rose Otto—10 drops
Lavender—20 drops

PMS Blend No. 2

Bergamot—20 drops   Lavender—10 drops
Clary Sage—15 drops

Painful Period Blend

Basil—10 drops   Eucalyptus—10 drops
Clary Sage—15 drops   Peppermint—10 drops

Irregular Period Blend

Basil—20 drops   Rose Otto—10 drops
Geranium—15 drops

Restarter Blend

Basil—15 drops   Rosemary—10 drops
Chamomile—10 drops   Rose Otto—10 drops

Hormonal Rebalancer

Basil—20 drops   Rose Otto—10 drops
Geranium—15 drops

All of the above are massage blends. Premenstrual syndrome can be greatly relieved by preventive care, and aromatherapy massage can greatly assist the regulation of menstruation. We will talk more about PMS, also known as premenstrual tension (PMT), and other experiences unique to the female body in the next chapter.

MIGRAINE

Basil, Lavender, Orange, Peppermint, base oil

Immediate Relief

Basil—1 drop   Peppermint—1 drop

Apply drops neat to the side of the head and massage into the temples.

Relaxing Massage Blend

Basil—15 drops   Orange—10 drops
Lavender—20 drops

To be used topically.

Relaxing Bath

Basil—4 drops   Orange—2 drops
Lavender—2 drops

There can be many contributing factors to migraine headaches. If pain persists, seek medical advice.

MISCARRIAGE
Geranium, Lavender, Neroli, Rose Otto, base oil

Body-Balancing Massage Blend

Geranium—20 drops   Rose Otto—10 drops
Neroli—15 drops

Soothing Bath

Geranium—2 drops   Neroli—2 drops
Lavender—4 drops

MORNING SICKNESS
See Nausea, Vomiting.

MOUTH ULCERS
Myrrh, Tea Tree

Ulcer Swab

Myrrh—1 drop   Tea Tree—1 drop

Two drops onto a cotton ball.

MUMPS

Chamomile (Roman), Eucalyptus, Lavender, tepid water

Cooling Bath

Eucalyptus—8 drops

Cooling Compress

Chamomile—1 drop　　　*Lavender—1 drop*
Eucalyptus—2 drops

MUSCLE ACHES AND PAINS

See Chapter 11.

NAUSEA, VOMITING

Fennel, Lavender, Peppermint

Travel Sickness Inhalation

Peppermint

Open the bottle of Peppermint oil and breathe in the vapors.

Morning Sickness Bath

Lavender—5 drops　　　*Peppermint—3 drops*

Relieving Vapors

Fennel—3 drops　　　*Peppermint—5 drops*

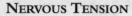

NERVOUS TENSION

Basil, Bergamot, Cedarwood, Geranium, Frankincense, Lavender, Neroli, Pine, Sandalwood, base oil

Calming Blend

Bergamot—15 drops   Neroli—10 drops
Lavender—20 drops

Soothing Blend *(nervous butterflies)*

Bergamot—15 drops   Lavender—20 drops
Cedarwood—10 drops

Restoring Blend *(long-term anxiousness)*

Basil—10 drops   Geranium—15 drops
Cedarwood—20 drops

Support Blend

Lavender—10 drops   Sandalwood—20 drops
Pine—15 drops

Fear-Release Blend

Frankincense—15 drops   Sandalwood—20 drops
Lavender—10 drops

These are all massage blends.

NEURALGIA

Geranium, Marjoram, Peppermint, Sandalwood, base oil

Nerve Swab

Peppermint—2 drops

Apply neat along nerve pathway (where you feel pain).

Massage Relief Blend

Geranium—15 drops   *Peppermint—10 drops*
Marjoram—10 drops   *Sandalwood—10 drops*

NOSEBLEED

Cypress

Inhalation

Cypress—4 drops

Prevention Swab

Add a few drops of Cypress to a cotton ball. Hold under the nose and sniff.

OBESITY

Fennel, Juniper, Lavender, Patchouli, Sandalwood, base oil

Massage Blend I

Fennel—20 drops   *Patchouli—15 drops*
Juniper—10 drops

Massage Blend II

Lavender—15 drops   Sandalwood—20 drops
Patchouli—10 drops

Alternate blends daily for four weeks.

PALPITATIONS

Lavender, Neroli, Ylang Ylang, base oil

Calming Blend

Lavender—20 drops   Ylang Ylang—15 drops
Neroli—10 drops

Use in macadamia nut massage base oil.

PILES

See Hemorrhoids.

RINGWORM

Lavender, Myrrh, Tea Tree

Medical Swab

Lavender—1 drop   Tea Tree—1 drop
Myrrh—1 drop

SCABIES

Bergamot, Lavender, Peppermint, Rosemary, Tea Tree, base oil

Antiseptic Blend I

Bergamot—10 drops   Tea Tree—15 drops
Lavender—20 drops

Antiseptic Blend II

Peppermint—10 drops   Tea Tree—15 drops
Rosemary—20 drops

Alternate blends daily for four weeks. These blends are to be applied topically and used in bathing.

SHINGLES (*Herpes Zoster*)
Clary Sage, Eucalyptus, Geranium, Lavender, Peppermint, base oil

Soothing Blend I

Clary Sage—10 drops   Lavender—20 drops
Geranium—15 drops

Soothing Blend II

Eucalyptus—10 drops   Peppermint—15 drops
Lavender—20 drops

Alternate these massage blends daily for four weeks.

SHOCK
Lavender, Neroli, Peppermint, Rosemary, base oil, hot water

Soothing Inhalation

Lavender—2 drops   Rosemary—1 drop
Neroli—1 drop

Massage Blend

Lavender—15 drops   Peppermint—20 drops
Neroli—10 drops

SINUSITIS

Eucalyptus, Lavender, Peppermint, Pine, Tea Tree, base oil, hot water

Relieving Inhalation Blend I

Eucalyptus—2 drops   Tea Tree—2 drops
Peppermint—2 drops

Relieving Inhalation Blend II

Eucalyptus—2 drops   Pine—1 drop
Peppermint—1 drop   Tea Tree—1 drop

Relief Blend

Eucalyptus—15 drops   Peppermint—15 drops
Lavender—15 drops

Use topically.

Massage Blend I

Eucalyptus—15 drops   Tea Tree—15 drops
Peppermint—15 drops

Massage Blend II

Eucalyptus—15 drops   Pine—10 drops
Peppermint—10 drops   Tea Tree—10 drops

SLEEPLESSNESS
See Insomnia.

SORE THROAT
Clary Sage, Sandalwood, Tea Tree

Throat Swab

Clary Sage—1 drop   Tea Tree—1 drop
Sandalwood—1 drop

Apply drops neat over throat area. Great for tonsillitis.

SPRAINS
Eucalyptus, Juniper, Lavender, Rosemary, Sage, base oil,
cool water

Massage Blend I

Eucalyptus—15 drops   Rosemary—10 drops
Lavender—20 drops

Massage Blend II

Eucalyptus—15 drops   Lavender—20 drops
Juniper—10 drops

Cool Compress

Eucalyptus—2 drops   Sage—1 drop
Juniper—1 drop

Alternate blends daily for four weeks.

STRETCH MARKS
Cypress, Frankincense, Lavender. See also Chapter 7.

Skin-Repair Blend

Cypress—5 drops   Lavender—25 drops
Frankincense—15 drops

STIES
Chamomile (Roman), distilled water (3 ounces)

Eyewash

Chamomile—2 drops ·

An infected boil or pimple on the eyelid can be painful and irritating. Use eyewash blend and cotton pads. Leave pads on for 10 minutes to soothe the eye.

TEETHING
Chamomile (Roman), Eucalyptus, Lavender, tepid water

Soothing Baby Bath

Chamomile—1 drop   Lavender—1 drop
Eucalyptus—1 drop

Disperse 3 drops into full baby bath, agitate the water, and bathe baby to soothe and comfort.

TONSILLITIS
See Sore Throat.

TOOTHACHE
Peppermint

Apply 1 drop of undiluted Peppermint oil to a cotton swab and dab onto the affected tooth. This is not to be used for babies or very young children. Remember, you should always consult your dentist.

TRAVEL SICKNESS
See Nausea, Vomiting.

ULCERS
Bergamot, Chamomile (German), Frankincense, Geranium, Lavender, Myrrh, base oil

Mouth Ulcer Dab

Myrrh—1 drop

Apply undiluted onto a cotton pad and place over affected area.

Peptic Ulcer Blend

Chamomile—15 drops   *Lavender—20 drops*
Geranium—15 drops

Use topically.

Skin Blend

Bergamot—15 drops   *Frankincense—15 drops*
Lavender—20 drops

Apply topically.

URINARY TRACT INFECTIONS
See Cystitis.

VARICOSE VEINS
Chamomile (Roman), Cypress, Lemon, Neroli, base oil

Topical Blend—General

Chamomile—5 drops   Lemon—10 drops
Cypress—20 drops   Neroli—10 drops

Use topically.

VOMITING
See Nausea, Vomiting.

WARTS
Lemon, Tea Tree, Thyme

Essential Swab

Lemon—1 drop   Thyme—1 drop
Tea Tree—1 drop

Apply with cotton ball twice a day.

WATER RETENTION
Cypress, Frankincense, Juniper, Rosemary, Sage, base oil, warm water. See also Chapter 6.

Massage Blend I

Cypress—10 drops   Juniper—15 drops
Frankincense—20 drops

Massage Blend II

Juniper—20 drops   Sage—15 drops
Rosemary—10 drops

Alternate blends daily for four weeks.

Bath Soak

Frankincense—2 drops   Rosemary—2 drops
Juniper—4 drops

WHOOPING COUGH

Basil, Lavender, Tea Tree, Thyme, base oil, hot water

Massage Blend

Basil—10 drops   Tea Tree—15 drops
Lavender—20 drops

Aromatic Vapors

Lavender—4 drops   Thyme—2 drops
Tea Tree—2 drops

WORMS

Bergamot, Eucalyptus, Fennel, Peppermint, base oil

Massage Blend

Bergamot—10 drops   Fennel—10 drops
Eucalyptus—15 drops   Peppermint—10 drops

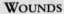

WOUNDS

Lavender, Tea Tree, distilled water (1½ ounces). See also Chapter 15.

Antiseptic Wash

Lavender—4 drops   *Tea Tree—5 drops*

YEAST INFECTION

Lavender, Tea Tree, Thyme, base oil, distilled water

Massage Blend

Lavender—10 drops   *Thyme—15 drops*
Tea Tree—20 drops

Douche

Lavender—2 drops   *Tea Tree—3 drops*

HEALED—AND NOT A DRUG IN SIGHT!

(Karen's Personal Experience)

From the time my daughter Rebecca was born (she is now a teenager), her life has embraced the healing vapors of essential oils. While we use them within our home environment daily, there have been two particular occasions when I have administered oils as an alternative to orthodox medicine, with astonishing results.

When Rebecca was just eighteen months old, I vividly remember her waking from a deep sleep in the middle of the night crying and with a very high fever.

As the mother of such a young one, I knew that high temperatures can be dangerous. I rang a doctor friend with a report of a temperature of 104 degrees. He advised me to give her aspirin immediately to suppress the fever and temperature, along with a good bath. Intuitively, this did not sound right to me, but to play it safe, I said I would keep in touch.

I prepared a large bowl of tepid water with 6 drops of Eucalyptus oil agitated across the surface of the water. I dampened several gauze cloths with the aromatic Eucalyptus water. I wrapped these around Rebecca's wrists and feet and laid one across her forehead, as well as wiping over the rest of her body.

The high temperature subsided almost immediately and was back to normal within thirty minutes while I continued to apply the cloths.

I have since used this remedy of Eucalyptus compresses on many sick adults and children with great success. So whenever there is fever, or high temperature, the feet, wrists, and forehead may be a good starting point for application of a Eucalyptus compress, or even a tepid Eucalyptus bath to soothe and disperse this condition, allowing the body's natural healing processes to occur.

As Rebecca grew older, her adventurous nature came to the fore. One day, when she was two and a half, we were playing on a beach and she wandered off and found a particular area to explore and build sand castles.

Three days later, her entire body was covered with red patches that were itching and weeping. I took her to a dermatologist, who advised me that she had contracted dermatitis from a particular type of sand.

I remembered—yes, the beach! He prescribed cortisone cream. I told him that I was an aromatherapist. A what? An aromatherapist, I repeated. I explained that I used only essential oils for treatment of the family first aid problems and believed in natural alternatives in preference to orthodox cures.

He said, a little disgustedly: "Look, lady, you can use what you like, but if this isn't cleared up, you'll have eczema on your hands with this child."

I went home with Becky and proceeded to make my own prescription of Bergamot, Patchouli, and Lavender in a base oil of avocado and wheat germ. Within four days, her skin was clear.

It was wonderful to see such positive results with my own daughter, working with the products I believe in. I have the utmost confidence in essential oils, and use aromatherapy as a first-line therapy in the treatment of most of the common ills and injuries that affect myself and my family.

6

Women's Special Needs

Cleanliness is next to Godliness.
　　　—John Wesley in Sermon 93, "On Dress"

SCIENCE HAS GONE to great lengths to discover the cycles of our solar system and of our weather—yet the biological cycles of a woman remain something of a mystery.

It has been estimated that 50 percent of women of reproductive age suffer from premenstrual syndrome (PMS) and up to 10 percent of these women suffer devastating symptoms that regularly make their life a misery. Dysmenorrhea (painful menstruation), postnatal depression, and menopausal problems are some symptoms that can be experienced by women and can make life tough and hard to cope with.

Our years of research and clinical experience with aromatherapy and the powers of the essential oils have convinced us, as well as many other researchers, that essential oils—in conjunction with careful dietary, lifestyle, and stress management—can help all women, no matter what their age, to a better quality of life. We believe that aromatherapy, which taps into the very essence of womanhood on a physiological basis, can greatly relieve—and in many cases completely eliminate—traumatic problems associated with many uniquely female disorders.

The great tragedy is that many women still do not know how the essential oils work and why they can be so useful in supporting us.

The fact is that the essential oils are akin to a woman's nature. We love to pamper ourselves, to accentuate our beauty; it's part of being a woman. The oils, apart from having a very sound therapeutic role to play, lift our spirits and can work wonders on our emotions. Our hormones are the most powerful chemicals in our bodies. They have the power to be physically and emotionally shattering, or they can make us feel wonderfully alive. We need to achieve a balance in our hormones, and aromatherapy can help us to find and maintain that center.

Once you start using the oils on a regular basis, your body soon begins to communicate with you. Your senses become more acute, decisive, and discerning.

Premenstrual Syndrome

Premenstrual Syndrome, or PMS, is a common problem among women today. The good news is that our research has shown conclusively that premenstrual syndrome can be alleviated—and quite often completely overcome—through the introduction of good lifestyle practices.

The essential oils play a crucial role here. They can work marvels in rebalancing our biological cycle. Working with the essential oils—in conjunction with good lifestyle practices such as a healthy diet, regular exercise, and taking care not to let stress get the better of you—will help you overcome the debilitating effects of PMS.

Many researchers have found that premenstrual syndrome is the result of an imbalance in the normal monthly hormonal cycle. Some say there are three definite phases in the monthly hormonal cycle of a normal woman, and these can be compared to the cycles of Mother Nature, such as the phases of the moon, the tides, and the passing of the seasons.

Following this analogy, if perchance spring and summer are too short, the earth does not receive its maximum sunlight, and the winter lasts too long, then the produce of the earth's soil suffers. Similarly, if the natural flow of female hormones is insufficient or ends too soon, the metabolism of many tissues and organs of the female body may be disrupted.

The role that aromatherapy can play in all of this is to help the body find a balance, and we can tell you that after working with these oils for many years, we believe there is no more effective way to bring the female body into balance.

Premenstrual tension can be addressed with self-massage blends for the week preceding the menstrual cycle. The following oils are most useful in PMS:

> *Cedarwood, Clary Sage, Fennel, Geranium, Neroli, Roman Chamomile, Rose Otto*

A combination of up to three oils can be selected, mixed into your massage base oil, and worn daily. One drop of each can also be dispersed onto a tissue and inhaled throughout the day.

We have had wonderful success using essential oils to balance our own cycles, and we have been able to help scores of other women to better harmony and health, too. Here's one story.

HOW MARY OVERCAME HER PMS WOES

Mary was 37 and had been happily married for 15 years. That was with the exception of her monthly "lows," during which life was tough on her household.

Mary and her husband had developed a unique arrangement. Three days prior to Mary's menstruation, her husband would pack his bags and leave home for "a long weekend." Three days of every month he took a break from his beloved wife. He stayed with family or friends, or arranged business trips.

The monthly "long weekend" was due to Mary's highly emotional mood swings, coupled with severe depression. They figured their marriage was perfect in between these down times. As soon as Mary's period commenced, her husband would move back in.

This pattern became a regular part of their life—that is, until Mary took action and visited our clinic. We suggested that she work with aromatic baths of Clary Sage, Geranium, and Rose Otto. One week prior to her period, we asked her to rub three drops of Clary Sage over her abdominal area with fast friction strokes, and repeat this once a day.

The first month came and went as normal. Her husband left as usual, and Mary reported only "slight emotional symptoms" on the first two days leading up to her period. On the third day, Mary rang her husband and invited him home for dinner. He returned and things were fine between them. They thought this was just a psychosomatic response to the treatment.

However, there was further improvement the following month, during which time Mary was able to keep control of her emotions. Hubby stayed at home for the first time. Three years later, he is still doing so.

We received a bunch of flowers three months after Mary's first self-treatment with aromatic oils, along with a note from her husband, which said: "Dear Clary Sage, Geranium, and Rose Otto, thank you for giving me back my wife!"

This was a wonderful healing story which we very much enjoyed being part of.

Dysmenorrhea

The first thing you must always consider when contemplating menstrual problems is that menstruation is not an ailment to be cured. Women are designed to bleed every month for a large part of their lives. However, the accompanying pain and discomfort can be greatly relieved with aromatherapy.

Some women have few problems with periods in an entire lifetime. Others suffer every month. Sometimes the pain is discernible only on the first days of a period. For others, the discomfort is so great they stop work and go to bed.

Clary Sage is the essential oil best known for its ability to ease dysmenorrhea. It is a hormone regulator and regular treatment can bring about a normalizing of the body's functions and an easing of pain.

Dysmenorrhea was first described as a medical disorder by the Father of Medicine himself, Hippocrates. His treatment was unusual, to say the least. It involved fumigation of the vulva with vapors of a concoction of sweet wine, fennel seeds, fennel root, and rose oil!

Other treatments have come and gone over the years. Most have been horrendously ineffective and others downright harmful to the human body.

WHAT CAUSES PERIOD PAINS?

In the 1950s, the frustrated medical community, seeking the source of PMS, turned to the theory of "psychological disturbance." Many practitioners today still are too inclined to throw difficult cases of PMS, dysmenorrhea, and post-natal depression into the "it's all in the mind" basket. We know, though, that at the end of each menstrual cycle, the fall in estrogen and progesterone secretion by the ovaries precipitates the shedding of the layer of cells lining the uterine cavity (endometrium), in the form of blood. This shedding is accompanied by the release of prostaglandins into the uterus and menstrual blood. In some women there is an excess of prostaglandins in the menstrual blood, and this can cause painful contractions of the uterine muscles.

Dysmenorrhea affects more than 50 percent of menstruating women. Even though suffering may be severe during menstruation, many women are reluctant to seek medical advice. Statistics show that fewer than 25 percent of women will visit a doctor about their problem.

So we would like to offer you a natural alternative to dysmenorrhea that we believe to be among the most effective treatments anywhere in the world. There are some very effective essential oils that can be used to alleviate period pains. The best oils are:

Basil, Bergamot, Clary Sage, Eucalyptus, Fennel, Geranium, Lavender, Peppermint, Roman Chamomile, Rose Otto

Painful Period Blend I

Basil—15 drops   Eucalyptus—10 drops
Clary Sage—10 drops   Peppermint—10 drops

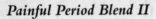
Painful Period Blend II

Basil—10 drops   Fennel—10 drops
Clary Sage—20 drops   Geranium—5 drops

Irregular Period Blend I

Basil—20 drops   Rose Otto—10 drops
Geranium—15 drops

Irregular Period Blend II

Basil—10 drops   Roman Chamomile—15 drops
Clary Sage—20 drops

Mix with a base oil and massage the abdominal area regularly.

Water Retention

Our general health plays a crucial role in determining whether we sufficiently eliminate waste liquids from our body. Water retention is a major concern for many women. Quite often, our weight can go up and down within days because our body isn't functioning properly and not eliminating fluids effectively.

Be sure to drink adequately during the day. Do not think that drinking water will add to your water retention problems. The reverse is more likely. The body is a smart biological system. Water retention is often a life-saving mechanism, especially during pregnancy. If you are dehydrated due to poor fluid consumption, your body will automatically store fluid until the drought is over.

Water retention can often be adequately addressed using specific essential oils. Juniper oil is a known natural and safe diuretic. Useful essential oils for the treatment of water retention are:

Cypress, Frankincense, Juniper, Rosemary, Sage

Water Drainage Massage Blend

Juniper—20 drops   *Sage—15 drops*
Rosemary—10 drops

In 3 ounces of base oil.

Bath Soak Blend

Frankincense—2 drops   *Rosemary—2 drops*
Juniper—4 drops

FURTHER TIPS FOR PMS

The following oils are also good for PMS conditions:

Bergamot, Cedarwood, Fennel, Orange,
Roman Chamomile

A full body massage with a combination of three oils is most effective. However, a lower back, chest, abdominal, hip, and buttocks massage can be effective as well.
Daily massage and daily bathing are important.

Postnatal Depression

After waiting nine months for your bundle of joy to arrive, it seems incongruous that severe depression can often follow childbirth. Studies indicate that mild postnatal depression (third-day blues) occurs in 50 percent of women, and long-term postnatal depression occurs in 5 to 10 percent of women.

The symptoms typically last only a few days, but some women find it takes many months before they feel like their old selves again. Fortunately, aromatherapy offers a very mild, effective, and harmonizing way to cope with post-baby blues. These essential oils are most effective in all cases of depression in women:

Basil, Bergamot, Clary Sage, Lavender, Neroli, Patchouli, Sandalwood, Ylang Ylang

See Chapter 5 for massage blends that can treat both acute and chronic cases of depression.

Menopause

The cause of menopause is failure of the ovaries. It is said that both ovaries have a limited active life span and that this is on average thirty-five to forty years. The word "menopause" simply means the stopping of cyclical menstrual bleeding, which occurs on average at fifty years of age (the normal range is between forty-five and fifty-five). There is a slowdown in ovarian activity with resultant hormonal imbalance for as long as five years before menstrual bleeding finally stops.

Unfortunately, during these years of hormonal change, many women feel generally unwell, physically and emotionally.

Once again, aromatherapy is the perfect complement to this time of change. Through regular use of the essential oils, we are able to bring about a marked balancing effect in the body. Many women who have taken on aromatic support to nurture themselves during menopause have dismissed their unpleasant symptoms and continued to live a vital life both physically and emotionally.

Useful essential oils for menopause are:

Bergamot, Clary Sage, Geranium, Roman Chamomile, Rose, Sage

You can use any of the above singularly, or make your-self a blend from the list. Alternatively, use one of the very effective blends in Chapter 5 for specific symptoms.

Yeast Infections

Yeast infections, also known as thrush, commonly afflict the vagina and can be most uncomfortable. A fungus called *Candida albicans* is the organism responsible. Symptoms are a white vaginal discharge and redness and itching of the vulva.

Tea Tree oil is gaining recognition around the world for its effectiveness in these fungal infections. Lavender and Thyme are other very effective essential oils for the treatment of this condition.

Massage Blend

Lavender—10 drops   Thyme—15 drops
Tea Tree—20 drops

In 3 ounces of base oil. Daily massage of the whole body with this blend for two weeks can bring about good results. If the condition persists, seek medical advice.

Sitz Bath

Lavender—2 drops   Tea Tree—3 drops

Beauty from Within

Throughout history, women have created beauty regimes and routines aimed at bringing about both a physical and and a psychological response in the body. These regimes were designed to nurture female emotions as well as improve the outward appearance. Certainly, true physical beauty comes from within.

Cleanliness and hygiene have always been the essence of female beauty regimes. Bathing has been the consistent theme throughout the ages: anointing the body with sweet-smelling perfumes and lotions together. The alchemy of blending and combining substances is intrinsically female. We love to make up concoctions and recipes. These talents are born within us and are enhanced as we travel the passages of life. Relationships, friends, children—generally speaking, we tend to feel better when we think toward and work in combinations.

Our female predecessors soaked and savored, indulged and created, knowing that they required time and attention to achieve desired beauty results. Of course, in today's fast-paced world, many women do not set aside hours upon hours to nurture their well-being, and we know from experience that quick pick-me-ups are of enormous value. However, you must always remember that the female body needs time to totally replenish and renew. We must harness the ebb and flow of our natural rhythm.

We suggest working with a varied beauty regime, from daily skin care to once-a-week activities to once-a-month full services. We also suggest a "four seasons" approach to women's health. Here are some suggestions to nurture your body beautiful.

The Deep Soak

Three times every seven days we suggest a relaxing/revitalizing deep-soak bath program. We recommend you soak in the evening before retiring, in the morning (on rising or after walk/run activity and/or meditation), then another evening bath. Spend 15 to 20 minutes at each soak. This routine softens the skin and rejuvenates the spirit. Warm to hot water is needed to revitalize, and body-temperature water is required for relaxation.

The Relaxing Bath

Bergamot—3 drops	or	*Orange—2 drops*
Cedarwood—2 drops		*Marjoram—10 drops*
Lavender—3 drops		*Sandalwood—2 drops*

The Revitalizing Bath

Basil—3 drops	or	Orange—10 drops
Frankincense—2 drops		Pine—2 drops
Lemon—2 drops		Rosemary—3 drops

Oils for the Four Seasons

WINTER

German Chamomile	Pine / Sandalwood
Lemongrass	Rosemary / Patchouli
Myrrh	Thyme / Eucalyptus

SPRING

Bergamot	Roman Chamomile
Clary Sage	Neroli
Fennel	Orange
Geranium	

SUMMER

Roman Chamomile	Lavender
Cypress	Peppermint
Frankincense	Vetiver
Juniper	

AUTUMN

Basil	Rose
Cedarwood	Tea Tree
Lemon	Ylang Ylang
Marjoram	

7

Skin Fitness

*Our skin is like a book—it tells a story. The
vicissitudes of life are written large across the page:
sadness, ill-health, stress and tension, crisis, dis-
aster, they are all there for the world to see.*
                          —Valerie Ann Worwood, London

A GLOWING, HEALTHY skin is fundamental to beauty.
Our skin is a living, breathing organ that needs to be
respected and well cared for. It is not mere vanity to
care for and be proud of healthy, smooth skin—just
common sense.

The skin deserves the best possible treatment, as it is
the part of the body that is continually exposed to the
elements and is most susceptible to damage from the
sun, housework, cooking, sports, and other activities.

Make essential oils part of your everyday skin care routine and you will have taken a mighty step toward ensuring that your skin is properly nourished. Add a few drops of essential oils to preparations such as hand creams, face cleaners, and moisturizers. This personalizes your existing skin care range and enhances its efficacy.

Essential oils are made up of molecules small enough to pass through the skin and into the body's circulation system. This useful attribute brings the therapeutic properties of essential oils to work quickly on the body through massage, bathing, or cosmetic treatment.

It doesn't take a lot of time or money to have a complexion that looks good, is free from blemishes, and is soft to the touch. All that is required is daily attention to cleansing and nourishing the skin. Nature's repair processes are slow and steady, with cells being constantly renewed. This renewal of cells happens very fast in young children, but begins to slow down as we get older. Slower cell renewal means that skin becomes drier, and wrinkles can appear; dead skin cells are shed more slowly, and the skin can lose its youthful bloom. By using the essential oils, we can aid in the body's repair processes and make our skin well nourished, vital, and glowing.

The removal of dead skin cells, by thorough cleansing and soaking with aromatic compresses each day, will also create a younger looking skin. It is the reflection of light from the skin that gives us a youthful complexion, and conversely, it is the accumulation of dead skin cells on an older skin that prevents this reflection of light, thereby giving the appearance of dull, aged skin.

It's so simple to create the reflection you wish to enjoy and radiate to the world around you. The following skin care program will show you how.

Your Face

From their adolescent years, women used to be taught to cleanse, tone, and moisturize the skin—a basic procedure to keep it glowing and healthy. As we grew older, we were instructed to increase our program to fully support the skin with heavier and richer night creams. This nightly regime could include an eye, throat, neck, and even a bust cream.

In our practice, however, we have developed a different kind of program to maintain skin fitness. It is based on a very basic principle: the skin does all its rebuilding during sleep and does not need "food," while during waking hours our skin needs nourishment and protection just like the rest of our body.

Take this example: On waking, we usually get the body moving and energized by taking in sustenance to maintain our energy. We clothe our body for protection. We continue to eat and drink during the day. By late evening, the body begins to slow down, preparing for sleep, and we are educated by nutritionists not to eat late at night as our body does not adequately digest food at this time. We certainly would never sit down to a heavy meal at two A.M. and expect our body to receive goodness from that food. Yet, in the quest for beauty, many imagine that these rich, heavy moisturizing creams will be digested capably by the resting body.

In our skin care program, on the other hand, we recommend that you keep your moisturizing and nourishing for the daytime, when your body is active in digestion and when your skin needs sustenance, moisturizing, and protection.

Since the skin is the body's largest organ, it should be able to digest anything that is used on it. And natural is always better.

Our program is designed to assist the skin in its natural elimination and rebuilding processes. Try it and see the difference. You will need to allow twenty-eight days for the skin to reestablish its own natural oil flow, but after this changeover period your skin will function far better than before.

MORNING PROGRAM

Step 1: Compress

Utensils: *water, basin, facecloth, gauze or cloth.*
Essential Oils: *Lavender, to soften and rebuild. Sage,
to cleanse and tone. Pine, to refreshen and oxygenate.
Frankincense, to rejuvenate.*

Fill a medium-sized bowl or half-fill a sink basin with very warm water (for more sensitive skin, use lukewarm only). Add 4 to 6 drops of your chosen essential oil and agitate the water surface. Immerse the facecloth in the water, and squeeze out the excess. Make sure the cloth is still holding lots of aromatic water, without dripping everywhere. While it's still very warm, place the cloth over the entire face and press firmly all over it, as if pressing the water into the skin. Repeat this at least four times.

Compressing the skin helps to tone and soften the skin. It also promotes the removal of dead cells and allows for a fresh, glowing skin. Just as we can remove the label from a bottle by soaking it in warm water, soaking or compressing the skin has the same effect on dead skin cells.

Step 2: Tone

Essential Oils: *Eucalyptus, to tone and invigorate. Orange, to soften and refresh. Tea Tree, as an antiseptic wash. Ylang Ylang, to regulate.*

Fill a small blue or amber glass bottle to about 3 ounces with warm water and add 3 drops of your chosen essential oils. Shake the bottle vigorously to disperse the oil. Using a cotton pad or your fingertips, smooth the aromatic water over the face—but not the eyes.

Step 3: Moisturize

Essential Oils: *Lavender, to assist regeneration of cells. Neroli, to strengthen broken capillaries. Sandalwood, to nourish and moisturize.*

To protect and nourish the skin, our favorite moisturizer is jojoba. Take a few drops of jojoba and add 1 drop of your chosen oil. Smooth over the face.

Apply a protective eye cream. We must keep our bodies guessing and not get into the habit of using the same products day in, day out. We recommend alternating your massage base oil between jojoba and peach kernel, and varying your essential oil combinations. You can easily add your essential oils to any of your existing skin care range of products to further enhance their functions.

In the Shower

A great way to awaken and energize the body is to take your blending bottle into the shower with you, with 4 drops of one essential oil in the bottle. We suggest Eucalyptus (to activate), Peppermint (to invigorate), or Rosemary (to stimulate). Add about 3 ounces of warm water once you're in the shower. Shake the bottle vigorously. Using a natural body brush, sprinkle the aromatic water over your body or your brush, then polish your entire body. This stimulates circulation and activates body and mind—we need to nurture both to act as a whole. Your skin will feel as smooth as silk. Once your body is dry, you can dress from your aromatic wardrobe. Follow the instructions in Chapter 4.

EVENING PROGRAM

Step 1: Compress

Essential Oils: *Eucalyptus, to activate and promote oxygen exchange. Lavender, to relax tired and tense skin; helps rebuilding. Lemongrass, helps to detoxify and tone the skin (2 drops only).*

Follow Step 1 from morning procedure.

Step 2: Cleanse

Use a natural cleaner and cotton, not tissues, to remove makeup. Remove eye makeup with cotton also. Do not use oils around the eye area.

Step 3: Compress Again

Step 4: Tone

Follow Step 2 from morning procedure.

Step 5: Leave Skin Free and Natural for Sleep

As previously mentioned, it takes twenty-eight days for the skin to go through its full rebuilding cycle. Be patient and allow the skin to begin functioning for itself again. The natural oil flow will take up where your night creams left off. If after twenty-eight days your skin feels dry or if you have mature skin, you can moisturize as a fifth step. But we recommend that you try to encourage your skin to function naturally.

Facial Massage

A once-weekly facial steam prior to massage can cleanse deeply, removing impurities. It's a good habit to get into. Using the inhalation method, steam the face and then proceed with the massage.

Our facial massage technique enables you to massage a partner or friend, or suitably give your own face a treatment. Begin by cleansing the skin, then use this procedure at least once a week.

The eye area should be well protected on the upper and lower lids with a suitable eye cream before applying the oil to the face. Prepare the area you have chosen by lying down in a comfortable spot and making sure that you are warm. Have your prepared oil nearby in a small bowl and place a headband around the hairline to protect the hair. You can do this massage standing or sitting, but you'll find it much more comfortable and relaxing lying down.

Begin by smoothing the oil over the throat and facial area, avoiding the eyes, gently stroking to cover all of the skin to the hairline. Begin at the collarbone, stroking upward along either side of the throat with alternating hands up to the jawline approximately ten to twelve times. Move under the chin and onto the facial area, with slightly separated fingers.

Now continue, with large, circular motions and slight pressure, over the cheeks and out to the hairline in an upward and backward movement. Move out to the earlobe and massage and gently stretch the lobe and outer ear area; move back onto the face, and place two to three finger pads on both sides of the nose.

Beginning at the end of the nose, using small, backward circular movements, work up the nose lightly, being careful not to squeeze the nostrils together, and up to the bridge of the nose. Using one finger pad on each side of the nose bridge toward the inner corner of the eye, apply a firm pressure three times, press and release. Lighten the pressure on the same spot and begin tiny, backward circular movements.

In a light, pinching action with the thumb and fingertips, move to the outer point of the eyebrow, gently pinching and lifting slightly as you slide along the line of the brow toward the temples. Assert a light pressure to the temple area. Press for a few moments and release three times. Using the finger pads of both hands, move to the forehead. Place the entire surface of the finger pads of both hands on the forehead, with the fingertips meeting in the center.

Alternate the hands, stroking upward toward the hairline eight to ten times. Take the right hand across to the left side of the forehead and place your four finger pads at the hairline. Your hand should be going across the forehead as if at right angles to the body. Now, with light pressure zigzag repeatedly across the forehead until you reach the hairline on the right side, using as much of the surface of the finger pads as possible.

Repeat with the left hand, moving from the right hairline to the left. Alternate hands as you repeat several times. Move more quickly each time.

Move the fingers into a vertical position on the forehead and, with hands meeting in the center, move out to the hairline by pressing the fingers into the surface of the skin in a rolling action of the hand.

Move to the cheeks, keeping the fingers in a vertical position, and, on either side of the nose, press into the surface of the skin with the finger pads, pressing and releasing in a rolling action out toward the hairline once again. Complete this pressing and rolling action six times on the forehead and cheeks, using as much of the finger surface as possible.

Using four finger pads, apply pressure down either side

of the nose, along the lip line and then along the chin, out along the upper jawline. Complete the massage with a few sweeping strokes.

Allow yourself time to relax and absorb the rejuvenating effects of the oil. If you wish to continue the treatment with a facial mask, take yourself to the bathroom and use a compress, submerging a cloth in warm or hot water and wrapping it completely around the facial area. Then press. Wipe clean. If you are not doing a facial mask, we suggest you blot any excess oil from your face by pressing over the area with a tissue. A thin film will remain, and in this way you will be using the oil to further moisturize and protect the skin.

_____ Warm Facial Mask _____

Utensils: *Oil warmer, essential oils, pastry brush, cold-pressed massage base oil.*

The skin has now been cleansed, steamed, and massaged. Once a week, you can also treat it to a delightful warm oil mask.

This mask will deeply cleanse and tone the delicate facial skin. An excellent way to apply it is with a natural bristle brush. We find a pastry brush is excellent. If the consistency of the mask is fine enough, it should easily glide onto the skin.

Using avocado or peach kernel as a base, take ⅙ ounce and warm it lightly in your vaporizer or over another source of heat. Add 2 drops of your chosen oil. Protect the eyes with an eye cream and lightly stroke the mask, moving out in sweeping strokes from the nose to the hairline, over the throat and facial area. Avoid the eye area. Have ready a small bowl with an infusion of chamomile tea and soaked cotton pads, so that you can refresh the eye tissue while you are lying down.

Leave the mask on and lie down for 10 to 15 minutes. Press firmly on the skin with a warm cloth to release any excess oil from the skin's surface. Leave a small amount of mask on the skin and lightly dust over with a natural powder (there are some powders available that are pulverized silk rather than talc). This will enable you to leave your treatment on without the skin looking too greasy.

To remove the mask, place a warm towel over the face to moisten the mask, then gently wipe it away.

Be sure all of the mask is removed before applying your moisturizer. Mineral water in your own spray bottle can be used to refresh and rehydrate the skin after any treatment, or simply throughout the day.

For particularly oily or blemished skin, this mask can be used twice weekly in the initial stages of treatment. For this type of skin, we strongly recommend a steam prior to the facial mask.

Your Body

CLEANSING

It is important to remember that before applying oils or creams of any type, the skin should be thoroughly cleansed to enable deep penetration. One suggestion is to use a natural bristle brush or loofah to shed any buildup of dead skin cells. We do not recommend dry skin brushing, as this is very harsh. Instead, rub the brush or loofah over the skin in the bath or shower. This can be done once or twice weekly.

Be sure to drink sufficient water to flush the lymphatic system. You might also look into your diet, cutting out or drastically reducing junk food intake, and perhaps cutting down also on stimulants such as alcohol, coffee, and extremely spicy foods—these all do the skin harm.

Facial cleansing is important morning and night. Read carefully our advice in the facial care section. Remember, it's best to avoid using soaps that create an imbalance in the skin's acid mantle, which is vital for protection against the elements.

Once the body, face, and hands have been cleansed, you are ready to begin using the oils on your skin.

DAILY MASSAGE

The first step is a daily body massage. This should prefer-ably be done in the morning. After emerging from the shower or bath, gently dry the skin, which will still be warm and extremely receptive to your chosen oil. Keep in mind it is always best to rotate your choice of oils for the skin on a daily basis. Every second day, you might want to massage a base oil alone into your skin to lubricate and nourish, and in this way you could experiment with the varying textures of the cold-pressed base oils. Avocado is one of our favorites. It may be that one day you would use avocado, and the next, olive. Always keep the body guessing.

Now to begin the actual massage. Starting at the feet, work over the feet and around the ankles, coming up into the calves, squeezing and stroking the muscles. Move to the thighs, stroking, applying firm pressure, and up to the buttocks, around and over to the abdominal area, working in a clockwise, circular motion, into the chest area and, for the ladies, cupping the breasts from side to side, alternating hands and working up toward the collarbone. Many people store a lot of tension in their pectoral muscles, and it is an important area to work with. Then, beginning at the fingertips, take advantage of the lubrication of the oils to push back the skin around the nails and the cuticles. Move up the forearm with light pressure and through to the shoulder.

These simple gliding strokes can be repeated several times to aid penetration of the oils. There should be no need to remove any oil before dressing. After a massage application of essential oils, it is important not to remove the oils for up to four hours. Wearing a fine sheen of oil will nourish and protect your skin throughout the day. You are now equipped to begin the day in a positive and powerful way.

Hand Care

To begin, soak the hands in a bowl of warm water with a few drops of Lavender oil from your basic kit. Gently dry the hands.

For the next step, which is your oil treatment, the oil can be warmed over a candle or on a heater in a small bowl before applying to the hands. See the recipe section later in this chapter for the blend of oils to use.

Once the oil is slightly warmed, take it into the palm of the hand and massage over the back and front of the hand and fingers, stroking the fingers from the hand to the tips, pulling and stretching each one.

Twist down each finger, drawing gently downward, applying a firm pressure. Press and release, sliding down the sides of each finger, and as you reach the tip, apply firm pressure to the nail and release. Massage between each bone up the hand toward the wrist, stroking with firm pressure.

Massage through the palm of the hand and onto the pad of the thumb, stretching out the hand gently but firmly. Now begin the massage treatment on the other hand.

When the procedure is complete, spend a little more time soaking, but this time in massage base oil combined with essential oils, not water. This may be a separate treatment altogether just for the nails.

Use a manicure utensil to push back the cuticles around the nails or, if this is not available, use a dry towel to apply gentle pressure to the cuticle area. If you are doing this treatment to nurture your hands in the evening, we suggest leaving the oil on overnight and simply wearing a pair of cotton gloves to bed. In this way, the contained body heat infuses the oil into your skin and protects your bed linens from the oil. Both the oil treatment and massage can be applied after and during an aromatic footbath also.

Recipes for Skin Care

We call our basic skin care regime our "maintenance program." Here are some recipes for daily use that can help your body repair and rejuvenate.

Lavender Yogurt Cleanser

20 lavender flowers *1⅔ ounces water*
5¼ ounces natural yogurt *5 drops Lavender*

1. Boil water.
2. Pour water over fresh lavender flowers. Let stand until cool; strain.
3. Blend yogurt with Lavender oil and lavender water. (To make lavender water, add 1 drop of Lavender oil to a 3¼-ounce (90-milliliter) blue bottle filled with purified or mineral water and let stand for 24 hours.)
4. Massage into skin. Rinse.

Antiseptic Wash
A gentle astringent for troubled skin

20 lavender flowers *8⅓ ounces apple cider vinegar*
1⅔ ounces witchhazel *5 drops Juniper*

1. Mix all ingredients together in a jar and seal.
2. Place in a warm area and let stand for two weeks. Remember to shake the jar every day!
3. Strain; apply to skin with natural cotton pad.

Varicose Veins

Cypress—5 drops   *Geranium—5 drops*

Combine these essential oils into ⅔ ounce massage base oil.

Cellulite

Cypress—7 drops   or   *Cypress—5 drops*
Rosemary—3 drops   *Juniper—5 drops*

Combine these essential oils into ⅔ ounce massage base oil.

HAND CARE

To ⅔ ounce avocado oil with ⅓ ounce peach kernel oil, add the following:

Normal Skin

Geranium—4 drops   *Sandalwood—4 drops*
Lavender—7 drops

Very Dry Skin

Bergamot—8 drops   *Patchouli—5 drops*
Frankincense—2 drops

NAILS

If you have brittle nails, use ⅓ ounce massage base oil—avocado or jojoba—and add up to 8 drops of Lemon oil. Massage into the cuticle area. This serves to nourish the nail bed, strengthening the nails.

FEET

Pour a small amount of water into a footbath and add essential oils, agitating the water before placing the feet in.

To Soothe Aching or Tired Feet

Juniper—3 drops   Rosemary—4 drops
Lavender—3 drops

For Perspiring Feet

Bergamot—6 drops   Lavender—2 drops
Cypress—2 drops

To Rejuvenate Feet

Clary Sage—4 drops   Rosemary—2 drops
Juniper—4 drops

Note: The oil treatment for nails can also be applied to the feet.

FACIAL MASSAGES

For all facial massages, use 10 drops of essential oil in ⅔ ounce peach kernel oil, or jojoba for oily skin.

For Normal Skin

Bergamot—1 drop   Sandalwood—1 drop
Lavender—1 drop

For Oily Skin

Basil—1 drop   Lemon—1 drop
Cypress—1 drop

For Blemished Skin

Cedarwood—2 drops   Cypress—1 drop

For Dry or Mature Skin

Frankincense—1 drop or   Geranium—1 drop
Geranium—1 drop   Sandalwood—1 drop
Lavender—3 drops   Ylang Ylang—1 drop

FACIAL STEAMING

For people with normal skin, a steam can be of great value. For people with sensitive skin or for those prone to broken capillaries, we recommend applying eyelid cream for protection with the facial steaming recipes.

For Normal Skin

Bergamot—3 drops   Geranium—2 drops

For Oily Skin

Cypress—2 drops   Lemon—2 drops
Juniper—1 drop

For Dry and Mature Skin

Geranium—2 drops   Patchouli—1 drop
Lavender—2 drops

FACIAL MASKS

Start with a mask base powder, which can be purchased at most pharmacies. We recommend fuller's earth or kaolin powder. Add to these distilled or filtered water to blend into a paste. Add 3 drops of essential oil to 1 heaping teaspoon of base powder. Add approximately 2 tablespoons of distilled water, making it into a fluid but consistent paste.

After cleansing the skin in the evening, remember to leave it free to breathe and rejuvenate during sleep. The essential oils to add for the facial mask are as follows:

For Dry and Mature Skin

Frankincense—1 drop   *Lavender—1 drop*
Geranium—1 drop

For Oily Skin

Bergamot—1 drop   *Juniper—1 drop*
Cypress—1 drop

For Acne or Blemished Skin

Cypress—1 drop   *Sage—1 drop*
Lemon—2 drops

Use this mask twice weekly in initial stages.

For Normal Skin

Eucalyptus—1 drop   *Lavender—2 drops*
Geranium—1 drop

Note: The facial mask for normal skin should not be used on extremely sensitive skin as it is quite stimulating and drawing. Avoid areas prone to broken capillaries. Those with dry skin can leave their mask on for five to ten minutes; oily skin, up to fifteen minutes. A further addition to these masks can be 1 teaspoon of honey, which is very nourishing to the skin.

Acne

When you have acne, remember that beauty is more than skin deep. What you see is an oily skin with a profusion of blackheads and pustules, and sometimes scarring, pitting, and inflammation. Acne occurs not only on the face but on the neck, back, and chest as well. The temptation to squeeze the spots and remove the infected pus is great; we suggest you refrain from doing this. Acne is very often the result of poor dietary and lifestyle habits, which leads to a hormonal imbalance and a condition known as seborrhoea—the overproduction of fat from the sebaceous glands.

Essential oil treatments, combined with a sensible diet, exercise, fresh air, and regular sunlight, often clear up the problem. Lymphatic flow is increased by the oils, allowing oxygen and other nutrients to reach the skin. The bactericide and anti-inflammatory properties of essential oils are extremely useful in helping the healing process. The relaxant properties of essential oils also play their part, as stress is a precursor of increased sebum production. We suggest that stimulants be avoided. Smoking can aggravate acne and pimples—a fact overlooked by many young people who take up smoking only to find that their skin pays a horrible price. Alcohol, coffee, tea, chocolate, and refined sugar–laden foods are other no-no's.

A useful massage oil treatment for acned skin (in 1⅔ ounces base oil) is:

Cypress—12 drops	or	*Bergamot—14 drops*
Lemon—5 drops		*Cypress—5 drops*
Tea Tree—8 drops		*Juniper—6 drops*

FIRST AID FOR SKIN

Lavender is the outdoor adventurer's savior, and is especially useful for campers to take away on holidays. It will alleviate the itch of mosquito bites and take the sting out of ant or other insect bites. Lavender can also be used on stinging nettle rash—and for any rash, for that matter. It is also great for sunburn, especially made up in a massage blend with avocado oil.

Tea Tree is a wonderful antiseptic. Use it neat on small infected areas. Tea Tree oil is also useful for gum diseases. Use 1 drop neat on your toothbrush or 3 drops in half a glass of water as a mouthwash. Tea Tree oil is good for inflamed pimples or in a mouthwash for mouth ulcers. (Chemically sensitive people should treat Tea Tree oil with caution.)

8

Care for Hair

Hair—it's our crowning glory.
—Rod Stewart, speaking to a News of the
World reporter in London

IT'S ONE OF the truly great beauty assets—a gleaming head of hair. The condition of your hair can really enhance your appearance. It can be a wonderful attribute that lifts your self-esteem—or an unruly afterthought that looks a mess.

A fortune is spent on hair products. Women in particular can spend the best part of half a day getting their hair cut and colored, yet many are still unhappy with the results. Many find their hair color fades quickly and looks dull.

We need a different strategy if our hair is really going to be our crowning glory!

The important thing to remember about hair is that it is there for a reason. Most of us tend to think of hair in terms of color, condition, and style, and forget that it also serves a purpose in protecting the scalp from extremes of temperature and regulating the loss of body heat from the head.

In many respects hair is similar to skin in that it reflects inner health. Each hair is made of the tough, stretchable protein called keratin, manufactured by the hair follicle—the same material of which fingernails are made and which is contained in dead skin cells.

The condition of a developing hair is largely dependent upon a good supply of blood, carrying adequate quantities of amino acids (the building blocks of protein), and vitamins and minerals, to the hair follicles.

Poor health, whatever its cause, leads to hair that lacks luster and life. An Australian scientist, Kenneth Seaton, has shown that there is an incredible relationship between the hair and the immune system.

"Damage to the hair can damage immunity," says Seaton, who has spent much time studying the relationship between hair, baldness, graying, and aging. "Similarly," he says, "damage to the immune system, and health in general, will always be indicated by a poor-looking head of hair.

"Striking evidence of this is that in any serious disease, hair loss is evident. Little wonder that lovely shiny, full, healthy hair has always indicated a healthy body."

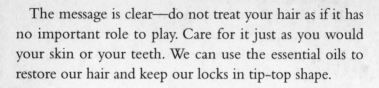

The message is clear—do not treat your hair as if it has no important role to play. Care for it just as you would your skin or your teeth. We can use the essential oils to restore our hair and keep our locks in tip-top shape.

Appearance

The color and length of our hair are invariably among the first identifying features mentioned when someone is talking about us. "You know, she's the one with long blond hair," or "the girl with shiny dark hair." It's not surprising, then, that we do spend so much time trying to get our hair looking good.

A good haircut is vital for anyone today, particularly if you are in the workforce or if you have to attend social functions where you need to look your best. There's no easy solution here, but it's best to find a hair stylist who will cut your hair to suit your face and body shape. Finding a style in a magazine that you like may be useful.

Make sure you find a stylist with whom you can communicate and who will work with you to find the styles that suit you best.

Color and tone are also important. Women have been coloring their hair for thousands of years. The Egyptians discovered henna as a natural lightener, and saffron and chamomile have also been used for ages.

Essential oils do not alter your natural hair color, but they can help to enhance it. Chamomile is effective in lightening blond hair. Sage, Rosemary, and Sandalwood are good for black or brunette hair, while Orange and Bergamot enhance red or ginger hair.

Bleached hair can also be helped by essential oil rinses. Essential oils are natural mediums that help rebalance the skin after chemical coloring of the hair.

_____ Hair Care _____

For hundreds of years, herbal preparations and oils have been used to improve the health and condition of the hair, to add luster and shine, to increase circulation, or to stimulate growth.

One of the pathways by which essential oils enter the body is via the hair follicles; therefore, hair treatments and rinses using essential oils are of great benefit to overall health.

While hair itself is dead, the vitality and condition of the scalp can be affected by chosen preparations, and the hair can be made to shine by using rinses. For example, Lemon essential oil will help rid the hair of residual alkaline after shampooing. This will make the hair shine with a natural luster. Sage used as a final rinse has been known to disguise the graying of hair. Massaging the scalp with essential oils will stimulate and encourage new hair growth and improve circulation.

In situations where it is not possible or advisable to wash your hair, a natural absorbent powder such as orris root brushed through it will absorb oil secretions. Follow with

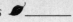

a few drops of Rosemary brushed through the hair to quickly restore a balance.

Damaged Hair

Hair can be damaged by many different things: the weather, perming, coloring, setting, bleaching, or even frequent washing with a strong shampoo. If your hair is damaged, lacking luster, or feeling dry, then a once-a-week warm oil treatment will replace vital nutrients, making the hair feel and look better, while at the same time feeding the scalp in which the hair grows.

Once you start to use essential oil treatments on your hair, you will see marked improvements in its texture and appearance.

Rinsing with Essential Oils

Fennel, Rosemary, and Sage can give dark hair luster and shine. Lemon and Chamomile can lighten and brighten fair hair. Add essential oils to water in a glass bottle. Seal well, shake vigorously, and allow at least twenty-four hours for the oils to be taken up by the water. Use as a final rinse to impart shine and luster to the hair and aromatize the head area, while providing a nourishing treatment to the scalp.

You will notice a marked difference in the way you feel after an aromatherapy hair treatment. Many people experience greater clarity, more energy, and a carefree feeling.

RINSES

Dark Hair

Bergamot—1 drop   Rosemary—3 drops
Geranium—1 drop

Fair Hair

Geranium—1 drop   Lemon—3 drops

Add these essential oil combinations to 1 quart water and shake vigorously before use.

TREATMENTS

Greasy/Oily Hair

Bergamot—12 drops   Lavender—10 drops
Cypress—3 drops

Dandruff

Cedarwood—3 drops   Eucalyptus—10 drops
Rosemary—12 drops

Damaged Hair

Geranium—5 drops   Sandalwood—10 drops
Lavender—10 drops

Loss of Hair

Juniper—7 drops   Rosemary—14 drops
Lavender—14 drops

Blend these combinations into a base of 1⅔ ounces of cold-pressed vegetable oil. Sweet almond is particularly good. Apply to dry hair and leave for about 20 minutes, wrapping head in a towel or disposable paper hair cover to maintain heat and aid penetration of the oils.

Note: When removing the treatment, shampoo must be added and worked through before any water is put on the hair. Wash thoroughly.

_____ Natural Hair Care _____

When taking a truly natural approach to hair care, it makes sense to avoid using harsh detergent-based shampoos. Go for a shampoo that claims to be mild, and see if it does the job. Make sure you don't stick to the same shampoo and conditioner week in, week out. It's our belief that we must always keep the body guessing. By using different essential oils in your hair-care treatments, you can challenge your hair to respond quickly.

Remember that milder shampoos are less likely to strip the hair of its acid mantle. Conditioners should be rich in proteins. To these products, you can add the essential oils listed under the category that best suits the present condition of your hair. This enhances the efficacy of your products and makes them personal to you.

If you have color or a permanent applied to your hair, the essential oils will enable you to offset some of the harmful effects of the chemical treatments. In this way, the oils will ensure that you won't fall victim to "hair today, gone tomorrow."

9

Sexuality and Sensuality

I don't think I have ever met a man or woman who is not turned on by perfume, of one kind or another. Smell is indelibly linked to sexuality. We can set the mood for intimacy and love making through aromatics.

— Brittania Hicks, News of the World

EVERY WOMAN IS a deeply sensual being with a need to be loved emotionally, intellectually, and physically. Unfortunately, this is not always achieved in relationships, and from our research and practical work with tens of thousands of women, we know that these unfulfilled needs can lead to mental and physical imbalances. Of course, men also need to be loved and cared for, and they too respond favorably, both physically and mentally, when their needs are being fulfilled.

A woman who is being loved deeply and sensitively usually appears happy, radiant, and relaxed. "She's glowing" is an oft-heard expression. From a physical viewpoint, our sexual responsiveness changes from day to day and depends on many factors. Mood, time of the menstrual cycle, hormone levels, general health, and the art, technique, and attitude of our lover are all important. Unfortunately, in today's fast-paced, often uncaring society, many women complain of dissatisfaction with their love lives. These women can develop deep feelings of disappointment and frustration, and this can lead to physical and emotional ill health.

One of the great attributes of the essential oils is their ability to stimulate and recharge our physical and mental states. We can use aromatics to alter our moods and emotions.

As we've discussed earlier, there are numerous studies that support the clinical experiences of aromatherapists, showing that aromatic stimulation can effectively bring about deep-seated emotional changes in our bodies.

The essences work on our physiology. They can uplift our spirits and help us rise above the irrational thinking that sometimes affects our emotional well-being. The oils can help us center our emotions. If we are to achieve our goals in life, we must have emotional poise. Only from this position can we truly be creative, peaceful, and happy.

_____ **Aromantics** _____

Aromatic oils can be used very effectively to create a mood for intimacy and lovemaking. When aroma and romantics come together, we have "aromantics."

Nothing is more stimulating to the senses than to return home after an intimate dinner for two and be greeted with the sensually stimulating aroma of Ylang Ylang or Rose Otto burning from your vaporizer.

With just a few drops of essential oil and a little imagination, you can give your love life a wonderful new dimension. Some of our clients have said aromatics helped them recharge the batteries in their sex lives. Certainly, the oils have been used very effectively to stimulate flagging sex drives in both men and women.

The alluring oils will help you to respond positively to your partner, and if you are both contributing to a deep-seated love and respect for one another, the essential oils can truly work wonders.

Certain essential oils have heady euphoric characteristics, so why not take your favorite and imbue your bedroom. Create an aromatic setting that will sweep you and your partner into a mood of sensual awareness and sexual excitement.

Rose, Patchouli, Orange, and Ylang Ylang are ideal for bedrooms and seduction. Rose is arguably the favorite perfume of all time and is an integral ingredient in many modern perfumes. (Cleopatra was reputed to have seduced Mark Antony by wearing Rose oil.) A drop of oil on a pillow or between the sheets can work wonders.

Aphrodisiacs

Certain essential oils have long been praised for their aphrodisiac qualities. One of the reasons they work so fast and effectively is that they act directly on the limbic portion of the brain, which is also responsible for sexual behavior and response.

In a less direct way, other essences possess the ability to spark fatigued reproductive glands into action, and so work to revive a waning interest in sex.

Study the sensuality blends and give your love life the inspiration and vitality it deserves.

_____ Sensual Massage _____

There is nothing more seductive than a good body massage, but many people refrain from using this simple technique because they do not know how to go about it.

Of course, body massage can be used simply for general health and to relieve stress. It can help tone our muscles and improve our circulation. It doesn't have to arouse the senses—that's all in the technique.

In Chapter 10 we will take you through a partner massage technique called "The Touch of Honor." We recommend that this massage be carried out free from sexual activity. But once you have learned the principles of massage, you can add your own special touch to create a truly sensual massage.

_____ Sexuality _____

Sexuality is intrinsically linked to health and beauty. When we make love, we become more aware of our bodies. To express your sexuality, you first must be able to know your body and be able to like it. To do this, you must take good care of your body.

Many women spend a lot of time taking care of their face, hands, and feet, "the bits that poke out." They cleanse, tone, and moisturize; they know every line and wrinkle. But more often than not, these same women know very little and care very little about the rest of their body.

It is even more important to study the shape and contour of your body than of your face, and to know the rhythm of your own body cycle.

With the greater awareness and education that we have available today, we can all be more confident in handling our reproductive system, knowing how to deal with menstruation, PMS, and mood swings. Our hormonal changes exist basically in three phases and are connected to our body expressions. From age eleven or twelve, women's breasts begin to develop, hips take shape, pubic hair appears, and the menstrual cycle begins. During our adult years, hormonal production is steady, then later in life we go through menopausal changes. All of these changes and cycles affect the way we look and feel, and ultimately the way we express our body and our sexuality.

By using your personally created essential oil blends on a daily basis (remembering to rotate the oils), you can learn to keep in touch with these changes as they occur, rather than looking in the mirror one day to be surprised by the form that stands before you. Feeling confident with your body can bring joy to your sexual expression and experiences. Rubbing oils over your body stimulates the senses. We can arouse our bodies, enabling us to become more responsive and enjoying the delights of aroma and touch simultaneously. We can become more sensual.

Pregnancy

Massage carefully during pregnancy, but most definitely do massage. Gentle caressing over the body is wonderful for the mother-to-be, while at the same time quieting baby-to-be inside. As the baby's weight increases, so does the pressure on the pelvis, the spine, the abdomen, and the legs—all very important areas to address with your aromatic wardrobe and daily body massage.

While it is particularly wonderful to receive a massage, it is most important to apply your oils daily to keep the skin supple and improve elasticity. Pay particular attention to the abdominal area, which is obviously where most of the stretching occurs. Ankles and legs can be supported and relieved by applying oils and also by soaking the ankles and feet in an essential oil footbath. (See Chapter 5.)

During Labor

This is a perfect time for the father-to-be to participate in the pregnancy. Massage the lower back with flowing, sweeping strokes from the back over the pelvic region and onto the tummy. A deep massage of the feet can help to take thoughts away from all the action in the abdominal area.

Wiping the forehead and face with a tepid aromatic

cloth between contractions helps to soothe and strengthen the birthing mother. Light strokes over the face with a calming oil blend help her release tension.

A vaporizer with its gentle candlelight can become a point of focus for the mother during labor. The slow release of soothing and restorative vapors warms the sometimes sterile hospital environment and can increase the loving connection between the parents-to-be.

After the birth, there is often a phase referred to as postnatal depression. We discussed this subject earlier in Chapter 6. This is a time to nurture and strengthen the body and spirit. Intimacy is needed and support is required. A loving massage with gentle strokes can be a way to reconnect sensually and intimately. More therapeutic and healing methods can be employed by massaging the abdominal and pelvic regions to help strengthen the natural functioning of the uterus as well as helping prevent stretch marks.

_____ Relationships _____

It is a great tragedy that love, for many people, is an ideal that is seldom, if ever, realized. We are told that love, like faith, can move mountains and overcome all obstacles. Yet even when some people are experiencing love, they can find it transient, fragile, possessive, often cruel—consuming itself with the very passion that triggered it.

For years, hand in hand with our work with essential oils, we have lived and studied relationships, and with the help of the aromatic experience, we have devised ways of strengthening them.

We believe relationships can be built on three fundamental structures: commitment, teamwork, and win/win. All aspects—communication, feeling, action—center around these three fundamentals.

COMMITMENT

Our commitments are held in place by our *word*. The very nature of feelings is that of change, so we always suggest that you hold on to the power of your word rather than surrender your word to feelings.

If you make a commitment to your partner via the spoken word, endeavor to honor that commitment, even if circumstances have changed since you made it. This, we believe, is fundamental to the success of any relationship. Take a moment to recall people you can trust and count on. Are they their word?

All actions occurring within relationships cost something—emotionally, physically, and spiritually. Rich relationships flourish when we clarify our position and commitment to each other. In this way, we can experience trust, safety, and freedom.

We know that aroma is linked to memory, so we can trigger reminders of loving exchanges and shared intimacy with special blends created with your partner. These we call "aromatic anchors"—enabling us to enjoy the freedom of self-expression within the canopy of our commitments.

TEAMWORK

Sharing strengths and working together are also major contributors to relationships. Making plans based on goals and projects that your partnership can achieve is a powerful way to get maximum benefits from a relationship. Together, you can achieve much more. By combining your talents, you will be stronger, more efficient, and more powerful in your daily affairs.

Just as each oil works individually, as a team they achieve greater results. Create your blends to empower and strengthen your efforts in teamwork.

WIN/WIN

Through conversation and honest communication, committed relationships work! Partners should feel free to be able to request and work within the framework of win/win, which means simply I win and you win. For instance, if your latest personal growth course or your aromatherapy course is going to contribute to your well-being, then hopefully your partner will accept that he/she too can win by supporting you in your new endeavor.

This is not about compromise. It's about resolution, and it produces powerful results by which you are able to jointly measure achievements—both personal and joint achievements.

This is a powerful contribution to success—a stimulant to increase self-esteem, energy (physical and emotional), and respect for one another. If the game of life is played with all players feeling as though they are always winning, self-expression, happiness, and achievement will be the result.

Aromatic Tools in Relationships

There are some wonderful aromatic techniques that can be adopted in relationships. These suggested techniques add real value and love to a relationship. In the next chapter, we will deal with massage, but here are a few other goodies.

THE AROMATIC FOOTBATH

This is wonderful to give and receive. It is essential to purchase a large stainless steel bowl, approximately 18 to 24 inches in diameter. Keep it exclusively for "feet treats"—either personal aromatic foot soaks while reading or watching TV, or to provide a perfect treat for your partner.

Fill the bowl to the three-quarters point with fairly warm water. Add 5 drops of your chosen essential oils. Our favorite reviver footbath blend is:

Rosemary—2 drops   *Tea Tree—1 drop*
Sage—2 drops

This is a great combination for reviving tired or sore feet. When your partner comes home, you can have the bowl prepared and offer a footbath. Many a woman has rolled up her husband's trouser legs and sat him down on a chair to delight him and help him unwind and release the tensions of his busy day.

The giver of the footbath gets to experience a wonderful aromatherapy inhalation and the receiver gets to experience bliss. The whole energy dynamic of one partner sitting at the feet of another—massaging and bringing pleasure to the other—has to be experienced.

The entire treatment can last as little as 5 minutes or as long as 20 minutes.

It is important when working with the feet to make contact with the *right foot first*. Allow the feet to be weightless in the water and massage under the water level. Move with firm, slow pressure in circular motions. Don't break contact with the foot until you complete the massage, then move to the left foot.

Make sure your own back is supported during the process. Keep it nice and straight, and have a towel on hand to dry the feet. Do all the lifting and moving for your loved one. Make the experience tender and caring—make it like the footbath you'd love to receive!

After drying the feet, massage in a warm oil blend or simply slip on a pair of wool socks.

THE AROMATIC NOTEBOOK

Get a small notebook and make it your personal notebook to each other. Place it in an easily accessible place where it can be spotted without difficulty and contributed to each day with a special word, verse, poem, or other message. For example:

> *11/11/96—I just want to thank you, darling, for all your wonderful support over the past few days. You have extended yourself to help me through. Thank you. Love, Judith Ann XXX*

The messages should always be dated, entered, and signed by the author. We suggest adding 1 drop of essential oil to each page. The fragrance is divine and enhances the mood of the message. Your notebook can become a beautiful keepsake for your relationship.

THE AROMATIC BATH

An aromatic bath is best taken with a partner; treating your friend to special pampering makes bath time fun. Of course, if you are single, you can enjoy the delights of an aromatic bath happily on your own.

Create the perfect ambience. Choose a blend of romantic essential oils or a combination to relax and revitalize. Bathing is truly an art form. You can enhance the mood with candles as your only source of lighting. Light your vaporizer and enhance the aromatic water further.

If you have a partner, seat yourself at one end and your partner at the other. You can massage each other's feet while chatting or simply enjoy each other in silence.

Make sure you have a washcloth each and a small rolled-up towel to support your necks if you intend staying in the tub for a while. Lean back and enjoy!

A good technique we recommend is to start with six candles for lighting. Wring out the washcloth and place it over your face. Take in some nice deep breaths to heighten relaxation. Keep pressing the warm cloth to your face—about five times. As you relax, blow out a candle—the light change further enhances relaxation. Blow out all the candles over the duration of your bath except one, which should remain the only source of light.

You can increase your sensual awareness by taking a small amount of massage oil (preblended for the occasion) and massaging each other when you are down to your last candle. This can turn the occasion into a very seductive bath. Choose oils that enhance intimacy.

Seductive Bath Combination I

Orange—4 drops   Ylang Ylang—2 drops
Patchouli—2 drops

Seductive Bath Combination II

Lavender—2 drops   Ylang Ylang—2 drops
Sandalwood—4 drops

You can make up a masculine combination:

Bergamot—3 drops   Sandalwood—3 drops
Frankincense—2 drops

Or a distinctly feminine combination:

Lavender—3 drops   Ylang Ylang—2 drops
Orange—3 drops

Relaxing Baths

The best way to use essential oils for an aromatic bath is to add them drop by drop once the bath is fully drawn. Make sure you are ready to climb in and that the doors and windows are closed so that you can take in the full healing benefits. Here are two of our favorite relaxation bath combinations:

Relaxation Bath I

Geranium—2 drops   Roman Chamomile—3 drops
Lavender—3 drops

Relaxation Bath II

Basil—2 drops   Cedarwood—3 drops
Bergamot—3 drops

When you wash your underwear, add a few drops of an essential oil to the rinse water. Your lingerie will smell fantastic, and your underwear drawer will smell wonderful when you open it!

Time and Effort

Just as a footnote to relationships, remember that the pleasure you get from a relationship depends largely on how much time you put aside to communicate and spend together. You don't need to spend every day together. Busy people with successful businesses can also have successful relationships. The secret is not so much spending a lot of time with your partner, but spending quality time together!

We believe it is vital in relationships to strengthen emotional bonds, to pamper your partner, and to bring pleasure to your loved one.

We can do this through our most primitive senses—touch and smell!

_____ Sensual Massage Blends _____

All in 1⅔ ounces massage base oil.

Aphrodisiac Blend I

Bergamot—5 drops   Ylang Ylang—10 drops
Rose—10 drops

Aphrodisiac Blend II

Bergamot—10 drops   Ylang Ylang—10 drops
Sandalwood—10 drops

Aphrodisiac Blend III

Clary Sage—5 drops   Patchouli—5 drops
Orange—10 drops   Ylang Ylang—5 drops

Bedroom-to-Boudoir Blend

Clary Sage   Patchouli   Sandalwood
Neroli   Rose   Ylang Ylang

Sensual Blend I

Neroli—10 drops   Patchouli—15 drops
Orange—20 drops

Sensual Blend II

Bergamot—10 drops   Sandalwood—15 drops
Lavender—20 drops

Sensual Blend III

Lavender—20 drops   Ylang Ylang—10 drops
Orange—15 drops

Sensual Blend IV

Clary Sage—10 drops   Orange—20 drops
Geranium—10 drops

Sensual Blend V

Bergamot—15 drops   Ylang Ylang—10 drops
Sandalwood—20 drops

Mix with generous amount of imagination. Optional extras: Soft music, low lights, vino.

10

The Magic of Massage

Massage should be a voyage of self-discovery, revealing how it feels to be totally relaxed and in tune with ourselves, to experience the pleasure of a body that can breathe, stand, and move freely.
—Lucinda Lidell, *The Book of Massage*

EVERYONE NEEDS TO relax, to escape the stresses of daily living. We can listen to music, observe the movement of clouds or the glowing of stars, sit on the beach and watch the waves or stroll along the shoreline searching for shells, watch the children playing in a park—these are all ways we inadvertently use to still the mind, to regain a sense of our own wholeness in the innocence of the moment.

As children, we climb trees and run around barefoot. We are at home with ourselves and our basic nature.

But as we grow older, we spend more and more time living in our heads. Throughout this book, we have been encouraging you to redress the balance. Now is the time to get back into your body. We have given you plenty of ideas on how to incorporate the essential oils into your life, to promote a greater sense of well-being.

Working hand-in-hand with the essential oils is the ancient art of massage. Massage is indelibly linked to aromatherapy, just as the sense of smell is linked to the sense of touch. Massage, like aromatherapy, can provide us with a means to counteract the relentless surge of work and domestic pressures. When everything seems too much, a good massage with high-quality essential oils can bring us back from the brink.

For thousands of years, some form of massage or laying on of hands has been used to heal and soothe the sick. To the ancient Greek and Roman physicians, massage was one of the principal means of healing and relieving pain. Once again, we look to Hippocrates, who wrote: "The physician must be experienced in many things, but assuredly in rubbing, for rubbing can bind a joint that is too loose, and loosen a joint that is too rigid."

We now know that rubbing—massage—can also do much more.

Don't Be Afraid to Touch

Massage is one of the oldest and simplest of all therapies. For pure pleasure and/or to bring about a relaxation response in the body, there is probably nothing better on this earth.

Yet it seems to be true that people today are afraid to touch one another. If you can break down the psychological barriers about touch, you will suddenly see and feel a whole new dimension open up to you.

One great advantage of massage is that it is nearly as pleasant to give as it is to receive.

Health Benefits of Massage

It has been scientifically proven that stroking a pet or another animal produces a relaxation response in that animal. Scientists have been able to show that a dog's blood pressure and anxiety levels can be substantially reduced simply by patting. Not surprisingly, stroking people has the same effect.

In the East, it is common for the healer to use his or her hands to bring about a healing response in the body. Unfortunately, mainstream Western medicine has overlooked massage as a genuine healing technique, although many modern-day doctors familiar with natural care techniques are correcting this lack.

Touch means contact, and is of vital importance to all human beings. It gives reassurance, warmth, pleasure, comfort, and renewed vitality. It tells us we are not alone. Touch is a language we all use to show our feelings, to demonstrate to others that they are loved, wanted, appreciated.

Massage can be stimulating or soothing, depending upon the speed and depth of your strokes. This is why it can make a person feel alive and ready for a sports session, or conversely, relaxed and sleepy. It can help relieve tension, soothe away headaches, relax taut and aching muscles, and banish insomnia.

If you haven't fully grasped our philosophy yet, then we need to point out again that this natural therapy—like most others—simply creates an environment for healing and regeneration. Massage, in conjunction with aromatherapy, can, we believe, help in the healing process of every acute and chronic disease known to mankind.

The body is a wonderful self-healing mechanism. Given the right conditions, your body will do its best to address the problem, whatever it may be. Of course, if the total load of your disease condition is too great, the body may not have the nerve energy required to restore the balance, and chronic disease may take root. However, you can still aid the recovery process and often relieve symptoms of your disorder through massage and aromatherapy. Keep in mind always that there are few shortcuts to good health. The more often you provide your body with the necessary care and healing environment, the more healing can occur. This goes for emotional healing as well.

Massage is simply any systematic form of touch that promotes comfort and a context for healing. Many times a client will tell us that they don't massage their partner or ailing friend, or child, simply because they don't know how. Yet they nearly always remember how they used to stroke their pet dog or cat. Massage is easy. Your instincts will lead the way.

So that you may have a better understanding of what you are doing, and to encourage you to develop your own valuable techniques, here are a few special methods of massage you may wish to employ.

_____ The Touch-of-Honor Massage _____

This is a special massage that establishes and maintains trust between couples. It rekindles sensory energy. Once you commit yourself to the principles of the Touch-of-Honor massage, you will learn to feel more secure with your partner.

We recommend that this massage be offered and received free of any sexual activity. It is good to make an appointment with your partner so that you can prepare for the event in advance. It also builds a sense of excitement and anticipation—an energy that both of you will enjoy being part of.

Of course, this massage—like any other—is best given and received with love and care. If you are not in a committed relationship, perhaps you have a platonic friend who would love to share your massage desires. It is, however, difficult to give yourself this particular massage, so try and find a buddy; you may be surprised how much better your friendship becomes.

Let us tell you about the Touch-of-Honor massage via one of our special clients, a delightful sixty-five-year-old man called Nigel. Nigel had been married to Mary for forty-five years. He came along to one of our workshops and we taught him how to do this particular massage. He thought it sounded great. He shared with us that he'd only ever touched his wife when they made love, or when they occasionally held hands walking, or during first aid. He was enthused by the massage techniques and wanted to offer something new to his relationship, which he believed had become regimented with time.

Nigel wrote an invitation to his wife and invited her to "an experience of a lifetime" at eight P.M. on Thursday evening. She said, "What on earth are you going to do with me?" He said: "I'm going to give you a massage, my darling, you'll never forget."

He made sure he had his equipment—essential oils, massage base oil, towels, sheets, blankets, soft music, flowers to decorate the room, a candle for light—he had it all!

At seven-thirty on Thursday evening, Nigel ran his wife an aromatic bath and asked her to soak for twenty minutes. He placed her robe and a towel to one side and asked her to pat her skin dry and to come into the room when she was ready. Mary kept looking at him with eyebrows raised.

Nigel had the room perfect. When she arrived, he had her lie facedown and covered her whole body gently with a sheet. He then uncovered her and massaged her back, neck, and shoulders and re-covered these parts. He massaged one arm at a time, making sure never to lose contact with the body during the massage. He covered her arms and tucked her in just like a child.

He worked on one leg, then the other, making sure not to massage too close to the genital area so as not to arouse his wife. He covered each leg on completion. He dislodged the covers and kept them over her body.

He gently whispered to her to turn over. He then massaged her face, neck, and chest—again making sure not to stimulate his wife by touching her nipples. He massaged her abdominal area in a clockwise direction, covering her again after each body part was massaged.

Mary was out like a light by this time, snoring gently. So Nigel covered her completely, except for her head, and went into the living room for half an hour to let his wife sleep.

Nigel surfaced at our shop a week later with a huge smile on his face. He told us that he had awakened the morning after his wife's massage to the smell of bacon and eggs and the song of a nightingale.

"Our relationship has been totally rejuvenated," he reported to us. "My wife said 'yes darling, no darling' for an entire week," he chuckled.

Nigel and Mary had rediscovered each other.

Nigel said while he had been massaging his wife he had reminisced about the girl he had married and recalled all that they had gone through together. He had made his wife feel special once more.

What Nigel had discovered, of course, was the subtle difference between sensuality and sexuality, and the wonderful, caring, and loving experience of touching.

We all deserve the magic of the Touch-of-Honor massage. Your partner will love you for it. Make it a special event.

_____ Back-to-Back Massage _____

This is a "mini-massage,"—a rubdown of your partner's back that can add value to each other's health and well-being.

In relationships, we really do "wear many hats." Playing the role of massage therapist once a week contributes to a healthy and vital relationship built on strength and wellness. We suggest scheduling a suitable time each week, a time commitment you keep even if it happens to fall in the middle of a disagreement. You may find that your massage makes you realize that the tiff was unimportant after all.

Prepare a minitreatment blend. You will only require ⅙ ounce per back massage. The recipes for all personal treatments can be chosen based on intuition, likes, and personal feelings. We suggest that this particular massage be done with a sloping back and neck and shoulder region—perhaps by having your partner kneel on all fours with the neck hanging downward (this is great for a 10-minute treatment). This position makes for easy massage of the tissue in those vital areas.

Otherwise, support the chest and abdominal area with four pillows—this allows the neck to fall forward relaxed and allows massage movements to be executed without any discomfort to your partner. You massage your partner, then your partner massages you.

The neck and shoulder area is where most people store tension. The neck muscles are always working, relaxing and contracting, even when we sleep. Our Back-to-Back massage is an ideal minitreatment. Of course, the obligatory blend of essential oils is needed to make it all worthwhile. The oils will help your body cleanse itself of toxins, and the manipulation keeps the muscles healthy, flexible, and toned.

Personally, we can reveal that rubdowns like the Back-to-Back massage have been a lifesaver in our own relationships at times. As we are both busy with our aromatherapy work, these massages stop us and center us. We learn to get back to basics—back-to-back!

_____ Carrying Out the Massage _____

An essential oil blend, care and sensitivity, a little time and energy, and a good pair of hands—that is all you need to begin practicing massage. There are a few points you should consider, however, when implementing your massages.

It is always best to set the scene in advance, so that you are well prepared for the massage session *before* you begin.

The room should be of even temperature, warmer in the colder months and cooler in the hot months. You will break the entire flow of the massage if you have to stop to go in search of some more oil, a heater, an extra blanket, or whatever. And you will defeat the whole purpose of the exercise if your partner cannot relax because he or she is chilly or hot or uncomfortable in some other way.

Think about your own comfort, as the giver, as well. To give good massage, you will need to be able to move freely, so comfortable clothes are a must. Make sure you continually check your posture; it is important that your back be flat, so keep the abdominal muscles pulled in tightly.

Central to the success of any massage are your state of mind and the state of mind of your partner. Before giving a treatment, prepare yourself mentally and talk to your partner to find out if there are any special problem areas that should be attended to.

Focus your energy when giving the massage. Remember that massage is a two-way flow of touch and response, a mutual exchange of energy. The hands, which both give and receive, and the skin—these are the instruments of communication during a massage. Relax, take your time, enjoy each caring stroke. Give the massage that you would like to receive.

The Basic Strokes

You will soon build your own language of touch once you start to massage on a regular basis, but it helps to have some idea of the basic strokes that experienced masseurs/masseuses use. Remember: always use the entire flat surface of your hands.

Gliding Strokes

Like waves rippling over rocks, these gentle rhythmic strokes glide over the skin. They are usually used on all parts of the body. The *long stroke* is the basic gliding stroke. Just let your hands float together along your partner's body. When you come to the limit of your natural reach, separate your hands and pull back along the sides. Circle around to repeat the stroke. *Feathering* is a brief, delicate stroke that brushes over the surface of the skin. It is mainly used to break contact gently, the strokes fading away like echoes of what has gone before. *Broad circling* is another gliding stroke. Move your hands in fairly wide circles, as if doing the breaststroke in miniature. This stroke can also serve to spread the oil more evenly over the body.

Medium-Depth Strokes

Following the gliding strokes, you can now start to work more deeply on the large muscle masses, using kneading, pulling, and wringing strokes. In all three strokes, your hands move in a continuously alternating rhythm, relaxing the muscles, draining away waste products, and aiding circulation.

Deep-Tissue Strokes

Deep and focused, these friction movements make use of thumbs, fingertips, or heels of the hands to reach right down into the tissue to where hidden tensions may lie. Having soothed and relaxed your partner with the broader, lighter, gliding and medium-depth strokes, you now penetrate below the superficial muscle layers or work around the joints with deep tissue strokes.

Percussion Strokes

These movements are stimulating rather than relaxing. They are performed repeatedly with alternate hands. Hacking, cupping, and pummeling with your fists or hands are all fairly noisy to apply, but have a marvelous regenerating effect. The main value of percussion strokes is to stimulate the soft-tissue areas, such as thighs and buttocks, toning the skin and improving the circulation. They are great before exercise! *Caution:* Do

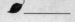

not massage over varicose veins. And always massage *toward* the heart.

_____ The Basic Massage Sequence _____

There is no hard and fast rule as to what areas of the body should be massaged first or last, but many experienced massage workers follow a basic sequence. This sequence is:

1. Back
2. Shoulders and neck
3. Back of legs
4. Arms and hands
5. Front of legs
6. Front of torso
7. Face and scalp

Of course, you may prefer to carry out your massage in a different sequence. The important thing is to make mental notes as to how your receivers respond and to act according to their needs and wishes.

It is vital to get the right blend of essential oils for your massage, depending upon the type of massage you are going to give and, again, the needs and wishes of the receiver.

_____ Working Surfaces _____

Working on a massage table is preferable; however, the floor or a bed can work just as well. Tables are often rather expensive, but they are a good investment if you are going to give and receive massages on a regular basis.

CONDITIONS TO AVOID

There are certain conditions that make massage inadvisable. These include skin eruptions such as boils or infectious rashes, inflamed joints, tumors, or any undiagnosed lumps, varicose veins, and cardiovascular problems such as thrombosis or phlebitis. Also, deep abdominal work during pregnancy should be avoided.

Massage Blends

Remember the basic rule for massage blends: a 1:2 dilution of essential oil to massage base oil. Use 10 drops of essential oil to every ⅔ ounce of sweet almond oil for general massage, or 5 drops of essential oil to ⅓ ounce of peach kernel oil for facial massage. When using up to three different essential oils, make sure your blend contains 5 drops total, not 5 drops of each essential oil.

Keep a special small mixing bowl to blend your aromatic delights, and always work with glass containers, never plastic. (Essential oils can actually pull the filler out of the plastic, which would then leach into the blend and adulterate it with plastic components. If you do use plastic, make sure that it's inert.)

Relaxation Blend

Bergamot—3 drops   Lavender—3 drops
Cedarwood—4 drops

Magic Moment Blend

Orange—2 drops   Sandalwood—4 drops
Rose—4 drops

Serenity Blend

Lavender—3 drops   Patchouli—3 drops
Orange—4 drops

Stress Buster Blend

Cedarwood—3 drops   Neroli—3 drops
Lavender—4 drops

Inner Cleansing

Juniper—3 drops   Rosemary—4 drops
Lemongrass—3 drops

Rejuvenation Blend

Frankincense—4 drops   Neroli—4 drops
Lavender—2 drops

11

Peak Performance

*Those who think they don't have time for exercise
will sooner or later find illness. When we make a
commitment to our health, we can reduce or eliminate the costs of supporting our diseases.*

—Judith White

STRENUOUS EXERTION IS no longer a natural part of
daily life. Millions of people in the West today spend a
third of their lives sitting in offices or behind steering
wheels. But the human body is designed for muscular
activity, and it does not function or maintain itself
properly without adequate exercise.

The easiest way to start on an exercise program is to
build some moderately strenuous activity into your
lifestyle. Set aside a few minutes most days to work

through some form of light exercise. Always warm up carefully first, especially if your surroundings are cold. Practice new movements slowly so as to avoid wrenching a muscle.

Most important, set yourself realistic goals! Don't overdo it on your first few days. You may be too discouraged to get back up next week. Remember, it is not how much exercise you do that really counts, but how regular and consistent you are. Once you build some aerobic fitness, you will be able to do a little more each time you exercise.

Exercise works hand in hand with the self-healing principles of aromatherapy. You don't have to pound yourself in the gym five times a week, or run six miles a day. You just have to get mobile and you will see the benefits. From an aromatherapist's point of view, exercise is essential if you want clear, vital skin and a healthy disposition. Exercise stimulates the lymphatic system, opens the pores, and clears debris from under the skin.

Our Rotation System

We believe one of the secrets of health and vitality is *rotation*. This means not allowing the body to get itself into a regular pattern. Patterns allow the body to establish routines that form a base for habits that can breed disease.

Our intrinsic nature is one of change. Health is not a static picture—it is ever-changing. We are beings of constant change. Therefore, we are at our dynamic best when we work with our own basic nature. We need to keep our body guessing. That way, we are not exhausting the same enzymes, hormones, and body systems.

We firmly encourage rotational activities in our clients's regular exercise programs. One day walking, another day stretching, another day a sports activity of some kind, and so on. A gym can provide you with regular, rotated exercise classes to add to your outdoor activities. If a morning walk is your choice of exercise, change the pace of your walk regularly—and take a different route. Remember, change is essential.

We have devised a wonderful exercise routine that works all body parts and is consistent with our theme of rotation. However, your personal exercise program will depend on your age and your level of fitness and agility. Use the regimen below as an insight into our theme of change and rotation.

Again, we stress that it is regular exercise that counts. The "no pain no gain" philosophy of the '80s is dead and buried, thank goodness. The new buzzwords in athletic circles these days are "balance," "exercise within your capacity," "listen to your body," and, here it is again, "rotation."

Stimulating essential oils can be used to boost circulation. There are some fantastic prewarmup blends that can motivate and stimulate. Certain essential oils are extremely valuable for postexercise rubdowns because of their ability to promote body repair.

Here are some aromatic ideas for incorporating the essential oils into your rotational exercise program. Give them a try; we know they'll make a difference to your

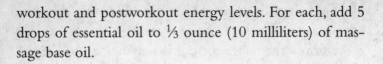

workout and postworkout energy levels. For each, add 5 drops of essential oil to ⅓ ounce (10 milliliters) of massage base oil.

The Aromatic Workout

MONDAY: Aerobic Class

With or without hand weights.

Before Class

Pine	Rosemary	Sandalwood

After Class

Frankincense	Lavender	Lemongrass

TUESDAY: Rest Day

For regeneration and balancing.

Cedarwood	Geranium	Orange

WEDNESDAY: Forty-five Minute Power Walk

Before

Eucalyptus	Sage	Tea Tree

After

Basil	Bergamot	Ylang Ylang

THURSDAY: Swimming or Tennis

Before

| Lemon | Patchouli | Peppermint |

After

| Juniper | Marjoram | Roman Chamomile |

FRIDAY: Rest Day

| Cedarwood | Neroli | Orange |

SATURDAY: Jogging, Cycling, or Step Class

Before

| Eucalyptus | Geranium | Myrrh |

After

| Cypress | Juniper | Vetiver |

SUNDAY: Jump Rope and Light Weights Workout

Before

| Lemongrass | Pine | Rosemary |

After

| Eucalyptus | Lavender | Thyme |

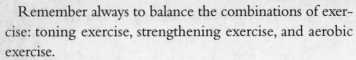

Remember always to balance the combinations of exercise: toning exercise, strengthening exercise, and aerobic exercise.

Be kind to yourself with exercise. There are a lot of self-styled fitness gurus in our society today who may not always give the best advice. Pace yourself, but be consistent. Make a commitment to yourself to exercise more frequently.

You will reap the benefits if you do.

Aromatic Blends for Sports Workshops and Athletics

Again, use 5 drops of essential oil to 1/3 ounce (10 milliliters) of massage base oil. All of these are massage blends.

ESSENTIAL OILS FOR MOTIVATION AND ENERGY

Citrus	_Trees_	_Herbs_
Bergamot	_Eucalyptus_	_Basil_
Lemon	_Sandalwood_	_Lemongrass_
		Peppermint
		Sage
		Thyme

Competition

Basil—30 drops   _Rosemary—10 drops_
Bergamot—30 drops

Endurance

Rosemary—10 drops   Thyme—10 drops
Sandalwood—25 drops

Motivation

Basil—15 drops   Lemongrass—15 drops
Eucalyptus—15 drops

Energy

Eucalyptus—10 drops   Sage—25 drops
Peppermint—10 drops

ESSENTIAL OILS FOR PHYSICAL SUPPORT

Florals

German Chamomile
Lavender

Resins

Frankincense

Trees

Cypress
Eucalyptus
Juniper
Sandalwood

Herbs

Lemongrass
Peppermint
Rosemary
Sage
Thyme

Respiratory

Eucalyptus—10 drops   Rosemary—25 drops
Peppermint—10 drops

Circulatory

Juniper—20 drops   Sage—15 drops
Rosemary—10 drops

Muscle Tonic

Eucalyptus—10 drops   Rosemary—25 drops
Lemongrass—10 drops

Joint Rub

Frankincense—15 drops   Juniper—25 drops
German Chamomile—5 drops

Relaxation

Juniper —10 drops   Sandalwood—15 drops
Lavender—20 drops

Muscle Energizer

Cypress—25 drops   Thyme—10 drops
Rosemary—10 drops

ESSENTIAL OILS FOR BODY REPAIR

Tennis Elbow

Cypress—25 drops   Lemongrass—10 drops
Eucalyptus—10 drops

Athlete's Foot

Lavender—25 drops   Thyme—10 drops
Tea Tree—10 drops

Locker Room Blend I

Eucalyptus—5 drops   Tea Tree—20 drops
Lemon—20 drops

Locker Room Blend II

Bergamot—30 drops   Rosemary—10 drops
Peppermint—5 drops

12

From Stress to Power

There is nothing either good or bad, but thinking
makes it so.

—*Hamlet,* Act II, Scene ii

MANY HIGHLY RESPECTED thinkers in various disciplines have concluded that thought—the mind—is the major determinant of how our lives will go.

Our futures are formed by the thoughts we hold most often and the words we speak. We literally become what we think and speak about. If we think and talk about how badly our lives are going, then, chances are, our lives will continue to be miserable. Conversely, if we look on the positive side of life, accept that life is not always going to be a breeze, and focus on the good things, we are likely to be happier and more content.

We are all aware of stress, every day of our lives, to some extent. We might see positive stress, of the type exercisers voluntarily put themselves under, or stress that comes from bickering with loved ones or running a highly demanding business.

*Dis*tress, however, is another thing altogether. This is when our stress becomes chronic, perhaps as a result of a series of ongoing events, with the result that we lose energy. Our love of life is traded for frustration and sometimes victimization. This is when the essential oils come into play, uplifting our spirits and centering our emotions.

Everyone handles stress differently. It must be addressed individually, and it never ceases to amaze us how the essential oils can help. We really do have healing and calming substances at our very fingertips—or noses, as the case may be. With our aromatic wardrobe, we can dress emotionally for every occasion.

We see the essential oils as our friends. They are there to service us 100 percent of the time. All we have to do is act to initiate the responses we desire.

The Stress Busters

Stress is a force that can strain and deform or renew and empower. The essential oils can truly help us calm our emotions, clear our minds, and focus more clearly on what we wish to achieve.

Next time you feel as though you are being pushed to the brink, that you can't cope with one more crying child, one more demanding phone call, one more bill to pay, one more nerve-racking day at the office—we invite you to inhale, bathe, or massage with some stress-reducing aromas and watch your tensions slip away.

We guarantee you'll be impressed with the results!

STRESS-REDUCING AROMATIC BATH PICK-ME-UPS

Bergamot—4 drops   *Lavender—2 drops*
Cedarwood—2 drops
or
Orange—4 drops   *Ylang Ylang—2 drops*
Sandalwood—2 drops
or
Bergamot—4 drops   *Patchouli—2 drops*
Geranium—2 drops

Depression

We sometimes need a little something to help when we are sad and troubled, to uplift our spirits and make us feel better about ourselves. We can use Clary Sage, or Rose Otto, or Ylang Ylang—together, singularly, or with other oils—until we feel once again in control of our emotions.

Breathing in the aromas of nature makes us feel more beautiful and tranquil, and helps us engage our inner strength to transform the worries of the day. The essences are one of God's gifts, and by inhaling their beauty, we can experience the joys of life.

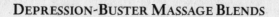

DEPRESSION-BUSTER MASSAGE BLENDS

Soothing Nervous Butterflies

Basil—8 drops   Lavender—17 drops
Bergamot—20 drops

For Chronic Anxiety

Cedarwood—17 drops   Lemongrass—8 drops
Lavender—20 drops

For Acute Anxiety

Geranium—8 drops   Sandalwood—17 drops
Lavender—20 drops

All in 3 ounces massage base oil. These formulas can be modified to create smaller massage blends, such as 5 drops of essential oil into ⅓ ounce massage base oil.

Making Your Own
Stress-Treatment Formulas

As you become more proficient with the essential oils, you can make your own synergistic blends to treat all types of ailments and emotional conditions.

For stress-related conditions, the oils can be used singly or in a combination of three. It helps to have a basic understanding as to which oils act, as a general rule, as stimulants and which ones act as sedatives or relaxants.

Stimulants

Basil, Clary Sage, Cypress, Eucalyptus, Fennel, Geranium, Juniper, Lemon, Lemongrass, Neroli, Peppermint, Pine, Rose Otto, Rosemary, Sage, Tea Tree, Thyme

Sedatives/Relaxants

Basil, Cedarwood, Chamomile (German and Roman), Frankincense, Lavender, Geranium, Marjoram, Myrrh, Neroli, Orange, Patchouli, Rose Otto, Sandalwood, Vetiver, Ylang Ylang

You will notice that some oils appear on both lists. This is because they are "adoptogens"—essential oils that act as natural balancers and instigate whichever reaction in the body is appropriate to achieve a state of homeostasis or balance.

Meditation

Just as regular physical exercise plays an important part in our lifestyle, so does emotional poise. There is no better way to still the mind and center our being than through meditation. Meditation, in conjunction with regular use of appropriate essential oils, is a most powerful antistress, antidepression therapy. We have seen chronically depressed individuals and people with very nervous, insecure dispositions completely rejuvenated through this process.

Meditation can be part of everyone's life. If stress is a

problem for you, you would do well to learn to meditate as soon as possible, and set aside a few minutes each day (up to 20 minutes twice a day) to practice it. We both meditate on a daily basis.

It is best to meditate in the mornings—upon awakening is ideal—and early evening. This helps you maintain your emotional state throughout the day and night. Many people believe meditation is only for "alternative types," but nothing could be further from the truth. More and more people are discovering the wonders of meditation and the joyous feelings of calm and control that come with it.

There are many different ways to meditate. As aromatherapists and lifestyle advisers, we suggest you ask around and see what technique feels good for you.

Meditation means stilling the mind. You need to sit quietly with your back straight—or, alternatively, lie on the floor—close your eyes, and still your mind by focusing on something. Popular focus points are breathing, a mantra (a word or saying that means something special to you), or mellow classical music. Creative visualization is an extension of meditation and can enable you to bring more positivity into your life. There are some excellent meditation tapes on the market today. Whichever way you learn to meditate, you can be sure that improved health will be one of the positive side effects of this wonderful therapy. Meditation helps throw off disease processes within the mind, emotions, and body.

MEDITATION RECIPES

Meditation I

Bergamot—5 drops   *Myrrh—2 drops*
Frankincense—2 drops

Meditation II

Clary Sage—4 drops   *Sandalwood—3 drops*
Frankincense—2 drops

Use in a vaporizer.

Breathing

Breathing is central to life, and breathing exercises can revitalize and recharge your body. You might like to refer back to Chapter 4 to see how breathing exercises can be incorporated into your lifestyle.

Some essential oils that promote improved oxygenation and respiration are:

Cedarwood—3 drops   *Tea Tree—2 drops*
Eucalyptus—4 drops

Eucalyptus—2 drops   *Peppermint—4 drops*
Lemon—3 drops

Lemon—5 drops   *Thyme—2 drops*
Tea Tree—2 drops

Experience these combinations in your vaporizer while practicing breathing exercises or simply focusing on deepening and slowing your breathing.

Psychoaromatherapy

Psychoaromatherapy is the term we give to the metaphysical benefits that can be obtained from using the essential oils. There is a strong relationship between the body, the mind, and the emotions—and, of course, our spiritual selves.

Blending various combinations of oils can produce specific effects. You must always keep an open mind and use what we call "aromatic listening skills"—observing each response and body-language signal and relating your observations to specific essential oils. This helps release judgments about the things you observe and increases your knowledge of the active components of each essential oil.

You should ask yourself the following questions whenever you use the essential oils for emotional advantage: (1) What would I like to experience from today's treatment? (2) How do I wish to feel physically, mentally, and emotionally?

Here are the oils that we know have a metaphysical-aroma association.

To Release Anger

Chamomile, Rose, Ylang Ylang

To Settle Anxiety

Basil, Bergamot, Geranium, Lavender, Neroli,

To Relieve Boredom

Basil, Frankincense, Peppermint

To Enhance Confidence

Cedarwood, Frankincense, Sandalwood, Vetiver

To Dispel Confusion

Cypress, Lemon, Rose

To Uplift Depressed Spirits

Bergamot, Clary Sage, Patchouli, Ylang Ylang

To Settle Emotional Instability

Bergamot, Geranium, Neroli

To Release Envy/Resentment/Jealousy

Rose, Juniper, Thyme

To Disperse Fears

Frankincense, Lavender, Sandalwood

To Relieve Frigidity

Chamomile, Clary Sage, Ylang Ylang

To Soothe Grief
Marjoram, Rose

To Relieve Insomnia
Bergamot, Lavender, Marjoram, Neroli, Orange

To Quiet Impatience/Irritability
Lavender, Neroli, Rose, Ylang Ylang

To Help Release Mental Fatigue/Poor Memory
Basil, Lemongrass, Pine, Rosemary

To Calm Nightmares
Bergamot, Frankincense, Sage

To End Distraction
Fennel, Sandalwood, Vetiver

To Reduce Stress
Bergamot, Lavender, Myrrh, Neroli, Rose, Sandalwood

To Heal Emotional Wounds
Chamomile, Rose

13

A Man's Choice

We have something really empowering for men here. The essential oils are far from being exclusively a female's domain.

—Karen Downes

NOWADAYS MANY MEN are stepping forward and making a more focused effort to be the best they can be—physically, mentally, and emotionally. More and more men are attending our aromatherapy workshops, and we are being invited to speak at a growing number of male-dominated business meetings. The essential oils have become extremely popular in the business sector as men and women alike look for ways to reduce stress and increase self-esteem and productivity.

Men are now turning to the essential oils and the

art of aromatherapy for improvement in their physical appearance and emotional stability. Many women find that they can easily introduce their partner to aromatherapy. Once men adjust to the natural aroma of the essential oils, experience the positive effects, and realize they are not solely for women, they are often thrilled with the results and become long-time users.

Many women may prefer to introduce aromatherapy to their man by letting him experience the healing and rejuvenating benefits of an aromatic massage. They may help him with some first aid tips using the essential oils, or give him a new aftershave experience. Men who have come into our clinic have reveled in the aromatic training and become proficient in the use of the essential oils for all sorts of things—including delivering the most wonderful massages to their partners and children.

Men can improve their skin care—they will look smarter and healthier—through use of the oils. Single men will see more heads turn their way when they use the oils to spruce up their appearance and give their body a pleasing, masculine aroma. Committed men in relationships will discover that their partners find them more appealing. And their self-esteem can be improved through use of the essential oils. As men begin to look better, they begin to feel better about themselves.

At our clinic, we don't have separate aromatherapy courses for men and women. Aromatherapy addresses life. The oils are equally effective for both sexes, although some oils tend to be favored by women and others by men.

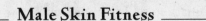

Male Skin Fitness

Who wants to kiss a man with flaking, dehydrated skin, shaving spots, and a rash? The essential oils can provide a lift for every man's love life. The oils are also effective in the workplace. A rough skin might not necessarily turn the boss off, but this is a competitive society and if stress and fatigue are written all over your face, your boss might decide to give the promotion or job to someone else— someone with a bright, clean, and healthy image.

Older men can be very attractive and sexy, provided they take care of themselves. Facial lines can add character. Neglect, on the other hand, shows a careless, perhaps lazy character, which can have adverse effects on a man's business and social dealings—not to mention the way he feels about himself from day to day.

Go for the best: the best you can personally be. Enhance your enthusiasm for life and communication. Increase your personal power, and live the abundant lifestyle you richly deserve with your new aromatherapy program.

The Male Starter Program

Step 1

Aromatic shower/body brushing. Sprinkle aromatic water over your body and brush all over as part of your shower.

Step 2

Aromatic body rub. Dress your body from your aromatic wardrobe with your daily massage blend.

Step 3

Preshave soak. Using hot water, Lavender essential oil, and your facecloth, soak and soften the skin by pressing and releasing a full, but not dripping, cloth on your face and neck. Repeat three or four times. This cleanses the skin and prepares it for shaving.

Step 4

Aftershave splash. Splash on a small amount of aromatic water to tone and soothe the skin after shaving.

Step 5

Regenerator. Add a vital nourishing glow by smoothing a blend of Lavender and jojoba over the skin to soothe and settle the skin. This blend protects the skin.

Step 6

Nightcap. Cleanse and tone, per the preshave soak, every evening prior to retiring.

Shaving

Shaving every day is like scraping sandpaper over your face. It can injure the protective layers of the skin and cause skin discomfort. Our aftershave splash is refreshing, antiseptic, and acne-clearing. We suggest you use it next time you shave.

Aftershave Splash

Bergamot—2 drops   *Tea Tree—2 drops*
Lavender—2 drops

Add to 3 ounces of distilled water.

Sensitive Skin Repair Blend

Bergamot—10 drops   *Sandalwood—15 drops*
Lavender—20 drops

Add to 3 ounces of jojoba oil.

_____ Balding _____

Hair is a touchy issue for many men. A man's self-image can be greatly reduced by baldness, and many dream of a magic drug that will restore the hair of their youth.

Basically, our genetic makeup determines how much hair we will lose as we age. Hair loss varies from person to person. Fortunately, the essential oils have proven quite helpful in reducing hair loss and improving the general health of the scalp. Remember, too, that the way we handle stress, shock, trauma, illness, and change can influence the degree of hair loss we experience.

Cosmetic surgery and new drugs and potions have helped stimulate hair growth and helped many men, but we believe the first step for all those concerned about hair loss should be to work with essential oils as part of a new

hair care program. Several of the essential oils can effectively stimulate atrophied hair follicles into producing hair
growth. And the oils—unlike chemical drugs—are harm-
less to the body if used correctly.

The essential oils won't work miracles, but they certainly
can help a great deal. It is important to realize that you will
be doing your hair a great service if you work on your
whole system with the essential oils—not just your head.

Essential Oils to Stimulate Hair Growth

*Basil, Cedarwood, Cypress, Geranium, Lavender, Neroli,
Rosemary, Sandalwood*

Use these oils singly or in a combination of three,
adding 4 to 6 drops to a bath or preparing a massage
blend to rub into the scalp. Warm oil treatments can be
applied up to four times a week during the initial six
weeks of the program and once a week thereafter.

Stimulation Blend

Lavender—15 drops   *Sandalwood—10 drops*
Rosemary—20 drops

Add 3 ounces jojoba oil as a massage blend, or combine
2 drops of each oil with 3 ounces distilled water for use
as a hair rinse each time you wash your hair.

The Male Genital Area

The essential oils can be of great help to male hygiene and
sexual health.

Antibacterial Wash Blend

Bergamot—2 drops   Tea Tree—2 drops
Lavender—2 drops

Add to 3 ounces tepid distilled water, agitate well, and bathe.

Anti-inflammatory Massage Blend

Bergamot—10 drops   Lavender—20 drops
German Camomile—15 drops

Add to 3 ounces jojoba oil.

Rejuvenating Massage Blend

Juniper—10 drops   Sandalwood—15 drops
Lavender—20 drops

Add to 3 ounces jojoba oil.

For the Working Man

MASCULINE AROMAS FOR HEALTHY EMOTIONS

Experiment with these blends as an "aromatic splash" to refresh yourself through the day, as well as part of your skin fitness regime. Incorporate combinations into your vaporizer and set the mood for a great work or home environment.

Relaxing Tonic

Bergamot, Geranium, Sandalwood

Nerve Release

Basil, Geranium, Lemongrass

Anxiety Relief

Bergamot, Cedarwood, Lavender

Nighttime Rejuvenation

Bergamot, Frankincense, Vetiver

Daytime Rejuvenation

Basil, Lemon, Rosemary

FOOT CARE ESSENTIALS

Foot Odor Dusting Powder

Sage—2 drops   Tea Tree—1 drop
1 tablespoon baking powder

This oil combination can also be used in a footbath.

14

The Working Woman

In the last decade there has been a marked increase in the number of men swapping traditional mother/father roles with their wives. That is to say, the women have gone off to work as the breadwinner, while the men have stayed at home to look after the children. It goes without saying that women really have made it in the workforce.
—Dr. Paul Aitken, Lexington Park, Maryland

IT IS A FACT of life that many men and women today spend far more waking time at their workplace than they do in the home with their families. Unfortunately, work for many becomes routine and tiresome, rather than a joyful challenge.

We encourage you to use the essential oils in your workplace, to set the mood of the day, to lift your spirits when necessary, and to create a wonderful, harmonious, and creative working environment. Remember that how we feel and think about our work can determine the stress we place ourselves under during our working day.

As Dr. Aitken, who studies behavioral sciences, has pointed out, these days more and more women are taking their careers seriously. And women are beings of rhythm. Our menstrual cycle alone tells us so. We need to be continually working with our body rhythms. Many of us power through the day to achieve our goals and ambitions, but we need to develop and keep in touch with all aspects of ourselves if we are to fulfill our true potential—physically, mentally, and emotionally. Listen to your body at all times and don't be afraid to act on intuition.

Being active women ourselves, we know all about being busy. We know about those inner thoughts and feelings that beckon us to contemplate all the things to do besides the ones we are presently engaged in. Listen to these thoughts, but don't act on them all. The modern working woman juggles many roles: she has to be a breadwinner, a wife, a mother, and a housekeeper as well. There are many tasks and activities to remember. We can often forget about beneficial little things, like our essential oil program, when the burden gets to be too much.

For this reason, it is vital that, when you introduce the essential oils into your daily routine, they be kept readily and visually accessible at all times, so as to "call us into action." I (Karen) remember deciding to make jogging part of my morning routine. But when that alarm went off that first day, I thought, "Just five more minutes." Needless to say, it was "goodbye, jog."

So the next day I placed the alarm at the other side of the room, so that I had to at least get out of bed to turn off the hideous ringing. In between my bed and the clock, I strategically placed my T-shirt, shorts, socks, and jogging shoes. That way, my equipment called me into action.

So have your aromatic equipment on hand to assist you throughout your working day. Don't wait until you get home to nurture yourself and to destress. You can regroup with an inhalation from a hot aromatic facecloth and by using your vaporizer to bring about a change in your environment.

Here are a few tips on how to charge, revitalize, and replenish your body and mind at the workplace.

At Work

On arrival, decide on the mood you want to establish for the day before you sit at your desk or start your activities. Arrive five minutes earlier, if you have to, so that you can light your vaporizer and create your aromatic blend for the day.

No matter where you work or what position you hold, you should ideally be able to create your own "aromatic sanctuary" at work.

Inspiration Blend

Basil—2 drops   Pine—4 drops
Bergamot—4 drops

Productivity Blend *(especially postlunch)*

Juniper—2 drops   Peppermint—4 drops
Lemon—4 drops

Mental Focus/Clarity Blend

Basil—2 drops   Rosemary—2 drops
Lemon—6 drops

Invigorating Blend

Eucalyptus—3 drops   Sage—3 drops
Lemongrass—4 drops

Joyful Communication/Creativity Blend

Bergamot—3 drops   Orange—4 drops
Frankincense—3 drops

To and from Work

No matter how you travel to and from work, you can use these techniques to influence your environment.

On a Tissue

Clary Sage—1 drop   Rosemary—1 drop
Lemon—4 drops

Inhale to keep alert and uplifted through the hustle and bustle. Also useful if you're feeling a little lethargic by midafternoon, take three deep breaths, counting to 5 both in and out.

Rub on the Dashboard

Lavender—2 drops   *Cedarwood—1 drop*

As the sun shines through the window, the warmth will vaporize the oils into the car. This is a great blend to soothe, calm, and dispense with anxiety or stress.

Over the Air Conditioner/Heater Duct

Position an aromatic tissue so that the air smells cleaner and fresher in your car during your drive.

In a Spray Pack

Keep this handy in the glove compartment or in your desk drawer at work. Add 2 drops of Bergamot to a small spray bottle (glass or stainless steel) of water. Agitate well. Used as an aromatic skin tonic and freshener.

As a Perfume

Use 2 drops of Rose Otto in jojoba oil on your pulse points.

_____ During the Work Day _____

Keep a washcloth handy in your desk drawer, handbag, or briefcase. At midday, take your washcloth to the bathroom and rinse it thoroughly under very hot water.

Add 2 or 3 drops of essential oil and squeeze any excess water from the cloth. Then hold it to your face and inhale deeply three times, in for a count of five and out for a count of five. This little regrouping will leave you feeling energetic and emotionally balanced.

Balance Mood Swings

Geranium—2 drops   Lavender—1 drop

Refreshen and Uplift

Bergamot—2 drops   Pine—1 drop

Stimulate/Activate the Mind

Lemon—1 drop   Rosemary—2 drops

Settle and Calm

Lavender—1 drop   Neroli—2 drop

Increase Energy/Activity

Eucalyptus—2 drops   Peppermint—1 drop

Alleviate Jet (and Other) Lag

Lavender—2 drops   Ylang Ylang—1 drop

15

Children's Special Needs

*Children—they can make our lives hell, but hell,
who would be without them?*

—Dr. John Kidd,
University of New South Wales

WHEN TREATING CHILDREN with essential oils, we
have to employ a sliding scale of dosage to mirror their
growth. Children respond brilliantly to the essential
oils and you should use them with confidence—
although some caution must be taken with the very
young. The pure essential oils are very powerful substances and you should keep dosages low when working with children.

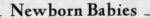
Newborn Babies

Newborn babies are particularly sensitive. The diluted essential oils can work wonders to clear up any troubles your baby may have in the first twelve months of life.

One of the gentlest yet most effective ways to treat various common baby ailments involves vaporization: allowing the molecules of essential oils to evaporate and circulate throughout the baby's room. Just place your vaporizer or a bowl of steaming water on the floor, well away from the baby, and add your essential oil so that it rises with the vapors and permeates the atmosphere. A quite adequate amount for babies is 5 drops of essential oil in the vaporizer, or diluted in 1 quart of hot water.

The following oils are the only essential oils we recommend for babies under twelve months. Each is to be used separately and always diluted when applied to the body.

Cedarwood, Chamomile (German and Roman), Lavender, Sandalwood

The Chamomile oils are great for soothing digestive disturbances, and are easily administered via vaporization. If your baby isn't sleeping well, use Lavender or Roman Chamomile. To freshen the air in the baby's room, use Lavender for its antiseptic and nurturing qualities.

Using even a tiny quantity of essential oil is infinitely better for your baby than commercial air fresheners, which usually contain harmful chemicals.

Useful baby blends include:

Diaper Rash Blend

Lavender—20 drops

In 3 ounces jojoba or olive oil. Apply to bottom each time diaper is changed.

Cradle Cap Blend

Cedarwood—20 drops

In 3 ounces jojoba or olive oil. Apply once a day.

Winter Protection Blend

Sandalwood—20 drops

In 3 ounces olive oil. Apply topically. This blend strengthens the immune system against colds and flu.

Restful Sleep Blend

Lavender—1 drop

Place on bedsheet 8 to 10 inches from baby's head.

_____ As Your Children Grow _____

The essential oils can be used as safe alternatives to pharmaceutical drugs in many cases of childhood illness. This is something that you as a parent will have to prove to yourself, but we encourage you to have confidence in the oils and the aromatic treatment of your children.

The essential oils work spectacularly in first aid. Children are constantly getting into scrapes of one sort or another. Bites and stings occur with monotonous regularity. The essential oils fight infection and promote healing—providing you as a parent with excellent first aid treatments. Many of the blends in Chapter 5, Health and Healing, are appropriate for children's ailments. Here are a few other blends that may come in handy for children four or five years and over.

Scrapes and Cuts Wash

Bergamot—2 drops   Tea Tree—2 drops
Lavender—2 drops

In 3 ounces distilled or filtered water.

Bruises Blend

Juniper—15 drops   Sandalwood—10 drops
Lavender—20 drops

In sweet almond massage base oil.

Burns Wash

Lavender—10 drops

In 3 ounces distilled or purified water.

Aches and Pains Blend (growing pains or cramps)

Lavender—20 drops   Orange—15 drops
Marjoram—10 drops

In 3 ounces sweet almond oil or macadamia oil.

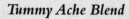
Tummy Ache Blend

Chamomile (Roman)—10 drops   *Peppermint—15 drops*
Lavender—20 drops

In 3 ounces sweet almond oil for massage. Adjust quantity for vaporization.

Nausea Relief Blend

Fennel—3 drops   *Peppermint—3 drops*

In vaporizer where child is resting. This blend can also be used when a child has motion sickness. Place 1 drop of each oil on a handkerchief or tissue and position it over the air vent of the car. Make sure the vent is switched to cool/outside air, and lower one of the rear windows.

Sleepy-Time Blend

Lavender—2 drops   *Sandalwood—2 drops*
Orange—2 drops

Use as a sleep-inducing bath. Or apply 1 drop of Lavender oil on either side of the pillow. This combination can also be used as a massage blend.

Head Lice Blend

Eucalyptus—15 drops   *Thyme—10 drops*
Tea Tree—20 drops

In 3 ounces of any massage base oil.

16

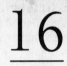

Celebrations and Special Occasions

YOUR VAPORIZER AND your aromatic wardrobe create a magical team. Together with your massage techniques and favorite massage base oils, you can achieve any effect you wish. We have come up with some popular essential oil blends to set the mood and provide the background for special occasions, holidays, or any particular moments you'd like to mark in a lovely and gracious way.

Christmas

An aromatic boost to the Christmas ambience.

Festive

Cedarwood, Geranium, Orange

Spiritual

Cedarwood, Frankincense, Lemon
or
Frankincense, Myrrh, Orange

Traditional

Myrrh, Orange, Pine

Valentine's Day

Sensual oils for Valentine's Day, or for setting a romantic mood any time!

Friendship

Lavender, Orange, Sandalwood

Lovers

Orange, Patchouli, Ylang Ylang

Pure Romantics

Lemon, Rose, Ylang Ylang

Easter

Enlightening

Lavender, Orange, Sandalwood

Renewing

Bergamot, Lavender, Lemon

Party Time

Relaxing Parties

Bergamot, Lavender, Sandalwood

Energizing

Bergamot, Lemongrass, Sage

Close Encounters

Clary Sage, Orange, Ylang Ylang

Special Ways to Use Your Oils

Vaporizers

6 to 8 drops

Fill the bowl at the top of your vaporizer with water. Add your drops of essential oil and light a long-burning candle to release the aroma.

Inhalation

4 drops

Fill a stainless steel bowl or basin with very hot (near boiling) water. Add essential oils, agitate the water, and place your head over the vapors, covering with a towel to keep the aromatic molecules enclosed. Breathe deeply and keep the eyes closed for two to five minutes.

Massage

1 drop per $\frac{1}{12}$ ounce (2 milliliters) of massage base oil

Using a glass measuring beaker, measure your desired amount of massage oil, $\frac{1}{3}$ to $\frac{2}{3}$ ounce, for a full body massage. Add your selected oils and mix to blend. The skin should not be greasy during an aromatherapy massage. It should be shiny and relatively dry to touch so all of the oils are absorbed.

Baths

6 to 8 drops

Add 8 drops of essential oil to a full bath. Agitate the water before climbing in. Keep door and windows closed to maximize the aromatic vapors. Soak for 10 minutes to take in the therapeutic value of the oils. Breathe deeply.

Shower

6 to 8 drops on a bath sponge

Wash your body as usual and follow by adding your chosen oils to a sponge or flannel and, with light friction, rub the oils over the entire body. This can replace the use of soap.

Foot Bath

6 drops

Using a large stainless steel bowl, half fill it with warm water. Add 6 drops of essential oil, agitate the water and soak the feet for 10 to 15 minutes. An ideal time for a foot massage to release tension is after work.

Room Sprays

10 drops to 1 quart water

Using a glass or stainless steel spray can, add 10 drops of oil blend to 1 quart of distilled water. Warm the water before adding the oil. Spray to freshen and cleanse the atmosphere, furniture, or carpets.

Lightbulbs

1 or 2 drops

Add your favorite essential oil to the bulb before it is turned on. Switch it on to let heat release the oil molecules. (Do not do this with a halogen bulb.)

Wood Fires

1 or 2 drops per log

Any of the woody oils will give a rich aromatic ambience to the warmth of wood fire. Allow some time for the oil to penetrate the wood. We suggest using Cedarwood, Cypress, Pine, or Sandalwood.

Sauna

3 drops per 3 ounces water

Add 3 drops of a cleansing, tonifying oil to a 3-ounce bottle of water and shake. Pour the aromatic water over hot coals. We suggest using Eucalyptus, Lemon, Pine, or Tea Tree.

Candles

1 drop

Light a candle and allow the wax to melt. Dispense 1 drop of oil into the liquid wax. The aroma will begin to rise. The essential oils are extremely volatile, so please be careful not to use directly on the naked flame.

Fragrant Flushes

10 drops

Use the spray method with a combination of 3 essential oils (10 drops total) to deodorize and freshen your bathroom. Spray several times into the toilet bowl after flushing.

Aromatic Ironing

5 drops

Disperse 5 drops of Lavender oil into a small glass or stainless steel spray can filled with water. Shake well and spray onto clothing or linens before ironing. Your shirts will smell delightful and your husband's shirts will remind him of you.

Fragrant Essentials

4 drops

Wash your delicate underwear in a final rinse of aromatic water. Place a cotton ball in your underwear drawer with your favorite oil combination.

Personalized Gifts

45 drops

Make your friends or loved ones a special aromatic massage blend for birthdays, Mother's Day, Father's Day, Christmas, Easter, or any other special occasion. We take a special oil blend to our hosts when we go to dinner parties. Give the blend an inspiring title: Breathe-Easy Blend (to relieve asthma and bronchial congestion) or Elle Macpherson Leg Blend (to address cellulite).

Aromatic Lipstick

½ drop

Dispense half a drop of essential oil onto the back of your hand and mix your lipstick and the oil with your lip brush.

Summing Up

Through the medium of "scentual awareness," we are dedicated to the promotion of personal growth and health and healing. By using aromatherapy, you can become more responsible for your health and well-being. We have lived and breathed aromatherapy for years and have seen our own lives transformed as a result of our commitment to this wonderful natural therapy. We invite you to join us on an exciting voyage of aromatic self-discovery.

We hope you gain from reading our book, and we hope it will act as a useful long-term reference guide as you explore the essential oils. These pages evolved from our commitment to remain educators in the aromatic field. The time and effort we put into the development and production of this book is our gift to you. Our book is packed with our own experiences, the experiences of the many clients who have passed through our clinics and workshops, and our extensive aromatherapeutic research.

We have an ongoing commitment to provide you with up-to-date information and professional advice, workshop and teaching programs, personalized aromatic prescriptions, and access to superior-quality aromatherapy products. Our contact address is listed at the back of this book.

Revel in the use of the essential oils. They are an expression of life.

Our book is presented to you with love and dedication.

—Judith White and Karen Downes

Bibliography

Literature that we have scanned over the years helped us considerably in the compilation of this book.

We extend our thanks and appreciation to the authors of these books and journals.

Aromatherapy

The Sense of Smell, Olfaction, Report by Dr. Lewis Thomas, Chancellor of Memorial Sloan-Kettering Cancer Center, New York, and Chairman of Monell Chemical Senses Center, Philadelphia.

The Book of Perfumes by Eugene Rimmel.

The Fragrant Pharmacy by Valerie Ann Worwood (Macmillan, London).

Aromatherapy for Women by Maggie Tisserand (Thorsons).

Using Essential Oils for Health and Beauty by Daniele Ryman (Century).

Scents and Scentuality by Judith White and Karen Day (Nacson & Sons).

The Relationship Between Health and Outside Stimuli, Report by Arch Minchin, Ph.D., University of Wisconsin, 1986.

Aromatherapy—Therapy or Placebo by Arch Minchin, Ph.D., Peter Young, Ph.D., University of Wisconsin, 1987.

Health and Fitness

The Biogenic Diet by Leslie Kenton (Arrow, London).

Peace of Mind by Ian Gawler (Hill of Content Publishing, Melbourne).

The Health Revolution by Ross Horne (Southwood Press).

Meditation by Judy Jacka (Lothian Publishing Company, Melbourne).

The Book of Massage, Lucinda Lidell with Sara Thomas, Carola Beresford Cooke, and Anthony Porter (Ebury Press).

The Family Book of Homeopathy by Dr. Andrew Lockie (Penguin Books Australia).

Nature and Health magazine, vol. 13, no. 1, February 1992.

Alternative Health Care for Women by Patsy Westcott (Collins Angus & Robertson Publishers).

Others

Blue Eyeshadow Should Still Be Illegal by Paula Begoun (Beginning Press, Seattle).

Index

About the Authors

Judith White and Karen Downes are expert aromatherapists who lecture on and teach aromatherapy throughout the world, with practices in Melbourne and Sydney, Australia. For more information about their workshops, seminars, and line of aromatherapy products, In Essence, you may write to: Wholistic Traders, 3 Abbott Street, Fairfield, Victoria 3078, Australia.

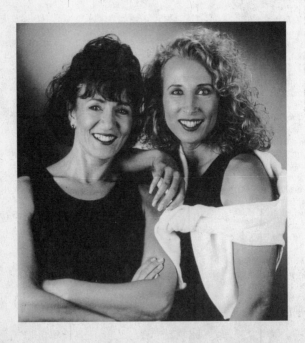